The Jossey-Bass Health Care Series brings together the most current information and ideas in health care from the leaders in the field. Titles from the Jossey-Bass Health Care Series include these essential health care resources:

*After Restructuring: Empowerment Strategies at Work in America's Hospitals*, Thomas G. Rundall, David B. Starkweather, Barbara R. Norrish

*Agility in Health Care: Strategies for Mastering Turbulent Markets*, Steven L. Goldman, Carol B. Graham

*Arthur Andersen Guide to Navigating Intermediate Sanctions: Compliance and Documentation Guidelines for Health Care and Other Tax-Exempt Organizations*, Diane Cornwell, Anne McGeorge, Jeff Frank, Vincent Crowley

*Breakthrough Performance, Accelerating the Transformation of Health Care Organizations*, Ellen J. Gaucher and Richard J. Coffey

*Creating the New American Hospital: A Time for Greatness*, V. Clayton Sherman

*Customer Service in Health Care: A Grassroots Approach to Creating a Culture of Excellence*, Kristin Baird

*Managing Patient Expectations: The Art of Finding and Keeping Loyal Patients*, Susan Keane Baker

*Technology and the Future of Health Care: Preparing for the Next 30 Years*, David Ellis

*Untapped Options: Building Links Between Marketing and Human Resources to Achieve Organizational Goals in Health Care*, Bea Northcott, Janette Helm

*Winning in the Women's Health Care Marketplace: A Comprehensive Plan for Health Care Strategists*, Genie James

# Remaking Health Care
# in America

. . . . . . . . . . . . . . . . . . . . . . . . . . . . . . . . . . . . .

Stephen M. Shortell
Robin R. Gillies
David A. Anderson
Karen Morgan Erickson
John B. Mitchell

# Remaking Health Care in America

## The Evolution of Organized Delivery Systems

### Second Edition

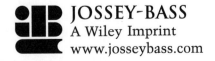
JOSSEY-BASS
A Wiley Imprint
www.josseybass.com

Published by Jossey-Bass
A Wiley Imprint
989 Market Street, San Francisco, CA 94103-1741   www.josseybass.com

Jossey-Bass books and products are available through most bookstores. To contact Jossey-Bass directly call our Customer Care Department within the U.S. at 800-956-7739, outside the U.S. at 317-572-3986 or fax 317-572-4002.

Jossey-Bass also publishes its books in a variety of electronic formats. Some content that appears in print may not be available in electronic books.

**Library of Congress Cataloging-in-Publication Data**

Remaking health care in America : the evolution of organized
delivery systems / Stephen M. Shortell ... [et al.].—2nd ed.
        p. cm. — (The Jossey-Bass health care series)
Includes bibliographical references and index.
    ISBN 0-7879-4823-3 (acid-free paper)
  1. Medical care—United States.  2. Health
facilities—Affiliations—United States.  3. Health services
administration—United States.  I. Shortell, Stephen M. (Stephen
Michael), 1944–    . II. Series.
  RA395.A3 R46 2000
362.1'0973—dc21

                                    00-008904

Printed in the United States of America
SECOND EDITION
HB Printing          10 9 8 7 6 5 4 3 2

# Contents

# Preface

· · · · · · · · · · · · · · · · · · · · · · · · · · · · · · · ·

In 1996 we published *Remaking Health Care in America: Building Organized Delivery Systems*, based on a systematic study of eleven organized delivery systems across the United States over a period of four years. Our book has been credited with laying the conceptual and empirical foundation for much of the integration work that has gone on over the past four years, not only in the United States but in Canada as well. We are, of course, pleased and gratified by this response.

Given the time and energy involved in the original undertaking, we had no intention of writing a sequel. We certainly maintain close, ongoing ties to most of the original study participants, but we also have turned our attention to other matters. Nevertheless, the issues, findings, and implications raised in our original book—regarding the need for more integrated delivery of care and less fragmentation, greater accountability, stronger linkages between health systems and their communities, and new ways of creating value—have been subjects of increased attention and controversy over the past four years. The performance of integrated health systems has been spotty, and the overall value of integration itself has been questioned. Growing consolidation among health plans, suppliers, and providers alike has led to increased levels of conflict among all parties. Overlaid on these developments, or, perhaps more accurately, as a result of these developments, has been a public backlash against certain aspects of "managed" care, the call for greater consumer protection, and the demand for greater public accountability from plans and providers alike. Further, the challenge of managing the multiple chronic illnesses of a growing elderly population increases at the same time that the country explores options for reforming the Medicare program. On top of all this is the growing recognition that the quality of health care in the United States leaves much to be desired for the poor and well-off alike.

Given these developments, we have received increasing inquiries regarding how our study systems are responding to these challenges. Are they "dis-integrating"? Are they financially viable? How are they now working with physicians? What is their experience in owning or not owning a health plan? Are they staying the course with their continuous quality improvement efforts? Are they finding new ways of creating value?

Finally, at the request of and encouragement by Andy Pasternack, Jossey-Bass Health Series Editor, and others, we decided that the time was right to revisit *Remaking Health Care in America*. Perhaps the old adage is true: books are not written; they are rewritten.

## Purpose and Approach

The purpose of this new edition is largely threefold: (1) to revisit the concept of an organized delivery system and the role of integration within that concept; (2) to provide an update on the accomplishments, failures, lessons learned, and future plans of most of the original study systems plus some of the experience of others not included in the original book; and (3) to explore the potential of the community health care management system concept for managing the health of individuals and communities, creating new types of value, and responding to multiple demands for accountability. To achieve these objectives, we draw on a wide range of data and information available from the systems, original data collection in a few selected areas, personal interviews, and analyses from several related studies. The secondary data include updates from each system's own financial statements, strategic plans, facilities and services offered, annual reports, organization charts, mission and vision statements, and related documents. Original data were collected on the extent to which leaders of each system believe they are achieving certain essential elements of an integrated health system; assessment of advances made in areas of functional, physician, and clinical integration; and measures of each system's involvement in community health improvement activities. These data and information were supplemented by telephone interviews that lasted between one and one and a half hours with key system leaders and addressed issues of functional, physician, and clinical integration, with emphasis placed on the barriers to and facilitators of success. In addition we drew on analyses and insights obtained from three related studies: (1) an examination of the relationships between physicians and health systems involving approximately fifty-five medical groups and fifteen systems across the United States (including five of the original participating study systems); (2) an evaluation of twenty-five community care networks (Bogue and Hall, 1997; Bazzoli and others, 1997); and (3) development of a taxonomy of health networks and systems (Bazzoli and others, 1999). Further detail on the data sources is presented in Resource A and further information on the study systems is presented in Resource B.

## Overview of the Contents

This book essentially follows the path of the original edition. Organized delivery systems are seen as the means to the end of maintaining and enhancing the health of individuals and communities. They are not the end in themselves. The goal is to discover ways of financing, organizing, and delivering health services in the United States (and, for that matter, in other countries) that lead to the creation of the greatest value for the consumer, recognizing that what individual consumers want may differ from what society as a whole may desire. The major focus of this book is on the organization and delivery elements, not the financing. But it is clear that the methods of financing and payment (recognizing that they are not the same) exert great influence on the methods of organization and delivery. The importance of aligning financial and payment incentives is underscored.

Chapter One highlights the need for a new framework for thinking about the health care system. It addresses issues of value and greater value creation and new demands for accountability. The growing importance of population-based community health improvement efforts is underscored.

Chapter Two examines the current research evidence and describes the elements of an ideal health system and assesses the extent to which organized delivery systems have achieved the ideal

Chapter Three provides an update on advances made in the areas of functional integration. Issues related to financial integration, human resources, strategic planning, information systems, Total Quality Management, and related functions are addressed. The importance of information systems and Total Quality Management is underscored.

Chapter Four examines the issues of physician-system integration and the advances that the study systems have made in this important area. This chapter draws on new work from related studies in addressing issues of governance and management of physician groups, compensation models, physician satisfaction, and the important role played by organizational culture.

Chapter Five addresses the issue of clinical integration—the extent to which services are coordinated across people, facilities, functions, and activities over time. Particular emphasis is given to the management of multiple chronic illnesses and the importance of developing linkages to the community. Factors associated with the successful implementation of new care management practices are also highlighted.

Chapter Six highlights changes and advances made by the study systems in their management and governance structures. It discusses the continuing challenge of overcoming the reliance on the hospital as a center of health care delivery and examines the progress made in creating cross-boundary, cross-functional management and governance roles.

Chapter Seven considers the future prospects for more integrated health care delivery and the role of the community health care management concept for addressing population-based health issues.

At the end of Chapters Three through Seven, we present brief cases from the study systems that illustrate some of the issues highlighted in each chapter.

## Audiences for the Book

There are four major audiences for this book: health services executives and clinical leaders; insurers and payers; health care policymakers at the local, state, and federal levels; and health services researchers. For health services executives and clinical leaders, the book provides practical suggestions and examples for developing organized delivery systems that can add value. Chapters Three through Six, dealing with issues of functional, physician-system, and clinical integration, as well as management and governance, will be of particular interest to executives and clinical leaders. For insurers and payers, the book's many examples, recommendations, best practices, and key success factors provide important criteria for contracting purposes, developing more effective payer-provider alliances, and accountability. Chapter Four, on physician-system integration, and Chapter Five, on clinical integration, will be of particular interest to purchasers. Chapter Seven provides lessons and ideas relevant to the future evolution of integrated health care and is likely to be of interest to all readers, particularly policymakers. For our health services research colleagues, the book provides an update on our earlier findings and refinement and extension of key concepts. We hope that all readers will at least skim Chapters One and Two, which highlight the major challenges facing our current health system, underscore the importance of population-based health care management, and review the evidence on the performance of organized delivery systems to date.

Creating organized delivery systems that can be used as a foundation for developing community health care management systems remains a challenging task. That it is evolutionary work is reflected in the experiences of the study systems. The experimentation and learning continue, although the barriers still outweigh the facilitators. We hope we have captured the most important lessons, clarified the real issues facing the integrated delivery of care, and provided some guidance for the future.

June 2000

Stephen M. Shortell
*Berkeley, California*

Robin R. Gillies
*Berkeley, California*

David A. Anderson
*Chicago, Illinois*

Karen Morgan Erickson
*Minneapolis, Minnesota*

John B. Mitchell
*Minneapolis, Minnesota*

# Acknowledgments

. . . . . . . . . . . . . . . . . . . . . . . . . . . . . . . .

This second edition of *Remaking Health Care in America: The Evolution of Organized Delivery System* would not have been possible without the cooperation of the study participants. System leaders and their staffs were generous in providing both time and materials. For their support, we thank system leaders Richard Risk, Advocate Health Care; Boone Powell, Jr., Baylor Health Care System; David Page, Fairview Health Services; Joe Wilczek, Franciscan Health System; Gail Warden, Henry Ford Health System; Judy Pelham, Mercy Health Services; David Bernd, Sentara Healthcare; Hank Walker, Sisters of Providence; and Van Johnson, Sutter Health. We also thank Lloyd Dean, Steve Derks, Charles Francis, Larry Majka, Scott Powder, and Lee Sacks, M.D., at Advocate Health Care; Joel T. Allison, John F. Anderson, M.D., L. Gerald Bryant, Carl E. Couch, M.D., and Lydia Jumonville at Baylor Health Care System; Gordon Alexander, M.D., Mary Cornils Baich, Don Berglund, Jim Fox, Dick Howard, Bill Maxwell, and Robert Meiches, M.D., at Fairview Health Services; Syd Bersante, Mike Fitzgerald, Jim Good, Dianna Kielian, Sister Anne McNamara, Mike Newcomb, D.O., and Laure Nichols at Franciscan Health System; Diana L. Kerr and Vinod Sahney at Henry Ford Health System; Louise Milobowski, Janet Pinkerton, Thomas Schindler, and Bruce Van Cleave at Mercy Health Services; Randy Axelrod, M.D., Richard Hill, Grace Hines, Rodney Hochman,

M.D., Douglas L. Johnson, Jenny Jones, Howard Kern, Sandra Miller, Irving Pike, M.D., Ken Rice, and Linda Thornhill at Sentara Healthcare; Claudia Haglund, John Koster, M.D., and John Lee at Sisters of Providence; and Jim Farrell, Pat Fry, Gordon Hunt, M.D., Cyndi Kettman, Bob Reed, and Elizabeth Shih at Sutter Health. G. Edwin Howe and Susan Buettner were generous in providing information regarding Aurora Health Care.

A special note of gratitude and recognition is due to John Troidl, doctoral candidate in health services and policy analysis at the University of California, Berkeley. John took the lead in overseeing the acquisition and summary of the study materials, conducted important telephone interviews, and wrote several minicases. The book would not have come together without his contributions.

Sherman Moore, Scott Walters, and Shannon Stokes from Hamilton HMC were instrumental in pulling together information for the book, especially for the management and governance chapter.

We recognize the helpful review comments of our colleagues Rob Burns, University of Pennsylvania; David Kindig, University of Wisconsin (Madison); Donald Light, Rutgers University; and Howard Zuckerman, University of Washington. Peter Grant and Gerald Hinckley from Davis, Wright, and Tremaine provided helpful assistance on legal issues, particularly involving gainsharing.

We benefited greatly from the manuscript preparation work of Alice Schaller and Pamela Barnes at the University of California, Berkeley. Thanks are also due to Andy Pasternack, Health Series Editor at Jossey-Bass, for his support and encouragement of this second edition. Finally, Dr. Shortell acknowledges the core support of the Blue Cross of California Chair in Health Policy and Management.

S. M. Shortell
R. R. Gillies
D. A. Anderson
K. M. Erickson
J. B. Mitchell

# The Authors

. . . . . . . . . . . . . . . . . . . . . . . . . . . . . . . . . . .

*Stephen M. Shortell* is the Blue Cross of California Distinguished Professor of Health Policy and Management and Professor of Organization Behavior in the Division of Health Policy and Management, School of Public Health, University of California (UC), Berkeley. He also holds appointments in the Haas School of Business, the Department of Sociology at UC Berkeley, and the Institute for Health Policy Studies, UC San Francisco. He is an associate of the Institute for Health Services Research and Policy Studies at Northwestern University. He is an elected member of the Institute of Medicine of the National Academy of Sciences and a Distinguished Fellow of the Association for Health Services Research. He is also senior adviser to the National Health Care Strategy Practice of Arthur Andersen.

Shortell received his undergraduate degree from the University of Notre Dame, his master's degree in public health and hospital administration from UCLA, and his Ph.D. in behavioral sciences from the University of Chicago.

A leading health care scholar, Shortell is the recipient of many awards, including the distinguished Baxter Prize for innovative health services research, the Gold Medal Award from the American College of Healthcare Executives, and the American Hospital Association's Honorary Lifetime Membership Award. He and his colleagues have received several Article of the Year and Book of the Year awards for their research.

*Robin R. Gillies* is a research specialist in the School of Public Health, University of California, Berkeley.

Gillies received her undergraduate degree in political science from the University of California, Irvine, and her M.A. and Ph.D. in political science from Northwestern University. Her background includes teaching, research, and administration. She has worked with Stephen Shortell on projects investigating the organization and performance of intensive care units, the implementation and impact of Continuous Quality Improvement/Total Quality Management on U.S. health care organizations, and the development of organized delivery systems. She is working with Shortell on studies of physician relationships with health care systems and the impact of physician organizations on the management of chronic illness.

*David A. Anderson* is a founding principal of Health Care Futures, a strategy consulting company dedicated to superior strategic thinking and implementation support for leading regional systems, academic medical centers, physician practices, and health care associations. As the partner in charge of the National Health Systems Integration Practice at KPMG, he helped lead the original efforts in the Health Systems Integration Study.

Anderson received his undergraduate degree from the University of South Dakota and his M.B.A. from the University of Iowa. He is a member of the American Institute of Certified Public Accountants. He has a wide range of experience working with regional health systems throughout the United States on strategic, financial, and capital planning; mergers, acquisitions, and divestitures; organizational and financial feasibility studies; and hospital closures.

*Karen Morgan Erickson* is a principal with Hamilton HMC, the health services division of the international management consulting firm Kurt Salmon Associates. She specializes in strategy development for a wide array of health care organizations, including health systems, academic medical centers, multispecialty group practices, community hospitals in both rural and urban areas, and physician-hospital organizations. In particular, she has experience in strategic planning, mergers and acquisitions, multiunit system integration, and service line planning.

Erickson received her undergraduate degree in biology from St. Olaf College and holds a master's degree in hospital and health care administration from the University of Minnesota. She held administrative positions at a major academic medical center, a community hospital, and a multispecialty group practice before joining Kurt Salmon.

*John B. Mitchell* is a founding principal of Health Care Futures. He specializes in the areas of strategic planning, mergers and affiliations, physician integration and practices management, managed care planning, and cardiovascular service development. He served as the engagement manager of the original Health Systems Integration Study and continues to conduct research on the effectiveness of health system physician integration and managed care organization performance.

Mitchell is on the faculty of the University of St. Thomas M.B.A. program and teaches at the University of Minnesota's Carlson School of Management. He received his law degree and master's degree in health care administration from the University of Minnesota. Prior to forming Health Care Futures, in 1996, he was a principal in the health care consulting practice of KPMG. He also had held positions in the acquisitions department of Allina and the University of Minnesota's legal department.

# Remaking Health Care in America

# 1

# The Search for Value and the Demand for Accountability

We began the first edition of *Remaking Health Care in America* by highlighting the harmful consequences of an unnecessarily fragmented health care delivery system. We suggested that the main reason for this fragmentation could be traced to the long-standing American value system emphasizing individualism over collectivism. We also suggested a need to balance individualistic values with those that promote a more collectivist orientation emphasizing solidarity and development of community. The relative imbalance between these two sets of values is at the root of our failure to make significant advances in increasing access to and use of needed health services and improving the quality and outcomes of care while containing the rate of growth of costs.

Building on these observations, we went on to discuss a number of building blocks for developing a sense of community and the role that might be played by organized health care delivery systems. We concluded, however, that "this requires a vision of what we want the system to do." We begin this book by revisiting this question.

## Wants, Needs, and Related Reflections

When it comes to health care, we want everything—convenient access, unlimited choice, good outcomes, and affordable costs—and we want it now. It is the American way. But what you want is not necessarily what I want, and neither of us may be really sure what "it" is we want because we do not fully know what "it" is. Most of us, most of the time, do not interact with the health care system. Rather, we have intermittent relationships that do not lend themselves to building cumulative knowledge. Although use of the Internet is changing the historical asymmetry of information between patients and physicians, it is often the case that individuals have difficulty separating their wants from their needs. Those of us with insurance coverage have the opportunity to reconcile this difference between wants and needs in our encounters with physicians and the health system at large. But for the approximately 45 million Americans without such coverage and millions more of the underinsured, this opportunity largely does not exist. In fact, at the collective level, the situation raises the following question: To what extent are the "wants" of the insured consuming so many of our health care resources that we cannot meet the "needs" of the uninsured?

## Value and Value Creation

We live in an extremely complex, pluralistic society where it is increasingly difficult to achieve consensus. In the effort to deal with the complexity, we often oversimplify by posing "solutions" in either-or terms. We need more inclusive ways of framing problems and challenges that permit us to consider the inherent complexity of the issues and choices in a meaningful way. We propose that value and value creation are two such concepts that enable us to consider many characteristics of desirable health care services simultaneously. The concept of *value* includes issues involving access, costs, use, service quality, technical quality, and outcomes of care. Value involves looking at the combination and interplay of these forces simultaneously. As consumers and purchasers, we seek organizations that for a given price can provide us with greater service quality, technical quality, and outcomes of care relative to other choices available to us. Or, conversely, for equivalent quality on the dimensions of interest to us, we will seek out organizations that can deliver the quality bundle for a lower price than other alternatives available to us.

*Value creation* encompasses the strategies, resources, and capabilities that an organization uses to meet the value preferences of its customers and stakeholders at large. The term *stakeholders* recognizes that health care organizations must do more than just satisfy those to whom they directly provide services.

Figure 1.1 shows a prototypical health care delivery value chain. The top row depicts the stakeholders that health care delivery systems must satisfy. It is important to note that each of these groups may value different outcomes with different sets of expectations. How value is created for individual patients, for example, may differ from how it is created for employers.

The second row depicts the desired end states and the row below that the competencies that produce the end states. They are competencies that range across the continuum of care. *Competency* is defined as a specific product or service that an organization can deliver to a specific group of consumers (Prahalad and Hamel, 1990).

The bottom row depicts the underlying capabilities of an organized delivery system that enable it to leverage its competencies. A *capability* is defined as a set of organizational skills and processes that support or leverage an entire value chain. These processes are inherently cross-functional (Stalk, Evans, and Shulman, 1992). Underlying capabilities are usually more difficult to achieve than are competencies and are therefore more difficult for competitors to imitate. Examples of underlying capabilities in organizations outside health care include General Electric's ability to manage change, 3M's ability to innovate through creative use of organizational design, Motorola's capabilities in total quality management (TQM), Wal-Mart's logistical support system, and Dell Computer's agility in reconfiguring its business units to adjust to rapidly changing market conditions. In similar fashion, the potential underlying capabilities of health care delivery systems reside in such functional integration capacities as their information systems and TQM processes, their ability to integrate physicians into systems of care, and their ability to achieve meaningful levels of clinical integration.

Figure 1.1. Value Chain of Health Care Delivery.

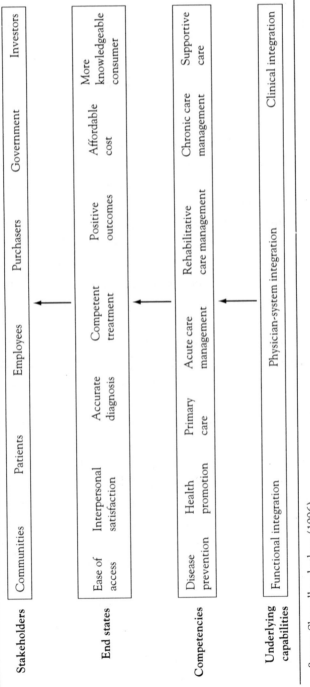

*Source:* Shortell and others (1996).

But at the beginning of the twenty-first century, we perceive that the entire value chain shown in Figure 1.1 is changing. In the past, value in the health care sector was created through investment in physical assets that led to the expansion of hospitals, the rise of academic medical centers, and the development of new technologies that required large physical settings for their placement. But with the ongoing concern over the costs of care, the ability of new technologies to treat more illness and disability on an outpatient and primary care basis, and, in particular, the information explosion represented by the Internet, value is migrating toward greater emphasis on these intangible assets. We believe that in the future, value will be created through greater investment in intangible assets: assessing customer needs and preferences, investing in one's employees and professional staff (the knowledge makers), and developing the knowledge-building capability of the organization (Mycek, 1998). As shown in Figure 1.2, this will require a redeployment of assets from the tangible box of bricks and mortar to investment in professionals and employees (human capital), information technology (knowledge capital), and the linkage of these to the customer-patient. This is a significant change involving the need for new strategic partners as well.

Figure 1.2. Redeployment of Health Care Capital from Tangible to Intangible Assets.

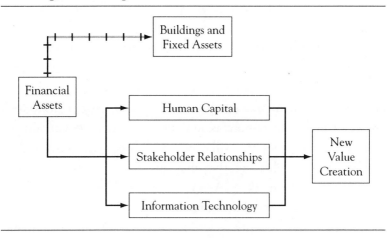

## Why Is This Shift Occurring?

In considering the end states shown in Figure 1.1, purchasers' dominant criterion in the value equation is still cost. Quality has historically been assumed to be approximately equal across providers because of intensive medical training, licensure, certification, and accreditation, and, in any event, it has been largely unmeasurable. However, significant progress has been made in measuring patient satisfaction (Cleary and Edgman, 1998; Cleary and McNeil, 1988; Wells and others, 1989; Carey and Teeters, 1995), the quality and outcomes of care (Schuster, McGlynn, and Brook, 1998), and documenting significant variations in clinical practice (Wennberg, 1999). This information is being drawn on by various purchasing groups and accreditation bodies, including the National Committee for Quality Assurance (NCQA), the Joint Commission on Accreditation of Health Care Organizations (JCAHCO), and the American Medical Association's Performance Committee (AMAP). In addition, local groups such as the Minnesota Buyers Health Care Action Group (BHCAG) and the Pacific Business Group on Health are implementing programs for increased accountability for outcomes of care. The Institute of Medicine Report on Patient Safety and Medical Errors provided a wake-up call for the nation (Institute of Medicine, 2000b). Although there is not yet a "business case for quality," that is, evidence of a positive impact on the bottom line, the evidence for building the case is growing.

We are also likely to see increased emphasis placed on quality and outcome criteria when we consider the dynamics of strategic competition between and among health plans and providers. As all plans and providers in an area strive to reduce costs, they begin to look alike on the cost dimension because their premiums are virtually the same. Over time, they also will begin to resemble each other in their benefit packages, although they may offer a wide array of packages for different niche markets. As a result, the only remaining dimension on which they can differentiate themselves is quality—both service and technical quality, as well as outcomes of care. As reliable, valid quality and outcome data are made more readily available to purchasers and the public at large, we can expect to see greater emphasis given in purchasing decisions to quality and outcome criteria. This is already occurring in Minnesota's Twin Cities area, where patient satisfaction data are beginning to influence choice of health plan and provider (Health Care Advisory Board, 1998).

These data are also beginning to reveal a hidden quality problem of large proportions in the United States (Schuster, McGlynn, and Brook, 1998). Compared to error rates in other sectors of the economy, health care fares poorly. Research reveals error rates of between 10,000 per 1 million opportunities for hospitalized patients injured by negligence to as high as 790,000 errors per 1 million opportunities in regard to eligible heart attack survivors who fail to receive beta blockers (Chassin, 1998). The clear exception is the reduction in number of deaths caused by anesthesia during surgery, which has fallen from approximately 50 per million in the 1970s and 1980s to the current 5.4 per million today (Ross and Tinker, 1994; Lunn and Devlin, 1987; Eichhorn, 1989; Orkin, 1993).

Nor do we fare any better when it comes to service quality. In a recent evaluation of different sectors of the U.S. economy, consumer satisfaction in hospitals was reported at 63 percent, tied at the bottom of the rung with police services and fast food restaurants, compared to a high of 85 percent for pet care and personal hygiene (Grant, 1998). In brief, on both service and technical quality dimensions, the United States has experienced significant value leakages for decades while being preoccupied with containing the cost of what most observers acknowledge is the most technologically advanced health system in the world.

## The New Value Frontier: Population-Based Health Management

It is likely that the next five to ten years will see considerable attention given to reducing variation and increasing the quality and outcomes of care as part of health care purchasing decisions. This is the immediate mountain that the health care system must climb, along with seeing whether it can figure out a political way of bringing approximately 45 million uninsured Americans along for the climb. But depending on the extent to which risk-based provider payment grows in various forms, there is an even greater value creation challenge ahead. This lies in recognizing the necessity of population-based health management involving disease prevention and health promotion in its broadest forms and the need for new strategic partners, from outside the organized health care delivery system, in order to realize the value inherent in such an approach.

Until everyone has a financial stake in promoting a healthy population, we will not achieve the health goals of the country as set forth originally in *Healthy People 2000* (U.S. Public Health Service, 1991) and its more recent update, *Healthy People 2010* (U.S. Public Health Service, 2000). Employers as payers, the federal and state governments as payers, the health plans, providers, and consumers must each bear some financial risk (as well as the prospect for financial reward) for restoring, maintaining, and enhancing one's health and the health of one's neighbors and the community in which one resides. Currently most of the financial risk is borne by the payer and health plans, with some evidence that risk is being transferred to providers through capitated and related forms of payment. There is relatively little cost sharing for insured consumers, and the uninsured are at full risk for their health problems.

Shared financial accountability for risk and rewards will establish the foundation for population-based health improvement. Once all parties are at risk for keeping people well, the importance of early prevention, health promotion, and community outreach efforts becomes obvious. Greater value is then created by intervening upstream in the value chain with disease prevention and health promotion efforts rather than waiting to fix the downstream problems of illness and disability. This shift will lead to an expansion of the mission of health care providers to include not only the provision of acute and chronic care but also to work with others in the community to produce a healthy population. As shown in Figure 1.3, this is how breakthroughs in value creation will be achieved in the future. One way of assessing value is to use quality-adjusted life-years (QALYs), calculated by multiplying the life expectancies by patient evaluations of their own health status in regard to mobility, self-care, usual activities, pain or discomfort, and anxiety or depression (Kind and others, 1994). Using quality-adjusted life-years (Robine and Ritchie, 1991; Robine, 1993; Kind, Gudex, and Dolan, 1994) as a metric of value and a surrogate for productive capacity, Figure 1.3 suggests that the acute care and chronic care business generally adds relatively little value. Primary care, with its focus on traditional prevention and early treatment, generally adds more value. And the greatest value is added by attacking the root causes of unhealthy behavior in the community reflected in substance abuse, crime, violence, and teenage pregnancy, which are related to air and water pollution, poor schools, inadequate law enforcement, fragile family structures, and lack of a social infrastructure. To address these issues, organizations must be in the business of not just providing health care services but of creating health, a radical departure from the past. Few health plans, individual providers, or health systems see themselves as being in the health business. They have neither the financial incentive, experience, nor capabilities to be in the business. But what if we paid providers for "producing" health? David Kindig (1997) has boldly laid out the logic for doing so and suggested a fifteen-year plan for achieving it. Significant advances in the ability to measure quality-adjusted life-years are being made (Siu and others, 1992; Gold, Franks, McCoy, and Fryback, 1998) and will continue.

Two other developments may also push us in this direction. The first is the extraordinary advances being made in the biomedical sciences, particularly in genetics and immunology. The implications of the Human Genome Project and related developments are immediate, and we are already entering the era of "predict, prevent, and manage" medicine (Goldsmith, 1996). These advances will enable

........................................

Figure 1.3. Value Creation by "Line of Business."

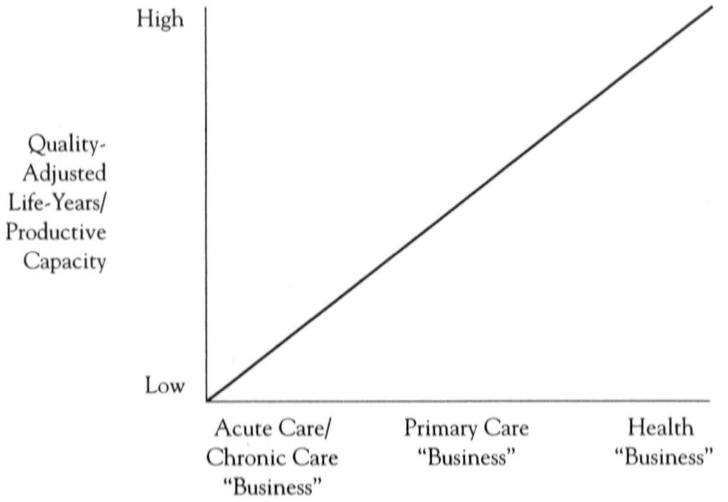

High

Quality-
Adjusted
Life-Years/
Productive
Capacity

Low

| Acute Care/ | Primary Care | Health |
| Chronic Care | "Business" | "Business" |
| "Business" | | |

us to identify genetic risks in individuals and populations and design both medical and social interventions either to eliminate or ameliorate the risk from evolving into major acute or chronic illness. As Goldsmith, (1996, p. 54) cogently states, "What this represents is movement from an event-driven to a risk-driven framework for health care payment. Instead of diagnosis and treatment as its principal business, our health care system will have to predict health risk and try to manage that risk before it flowers into illness and cost."

This will require a much closer interface between the biomedical and the behavioral and social sciences in order to achieve a greater understanding of how community and social factors influence disease and disability (Evans, Barer, and Marmor, 1994; Wilkinson, Kawachi, and Kennedy, 1998). These developments will raise a variety of legal, moral, and ethical issues. For example, employers may discriminate against those with "predicted" illness, and health plans may decide not to insure them. This, of course, is an extension of the argument that no health plan and no employer wants to be burdened with a disproportionate share of high-risk individuals. The argument is also made that current methods of risk adjustment are inadequate to deal with the problem. But this is ironic in the era of "predict and prevent" medicine because such advanced knowledge represents the perfect risk adjuster. By knowing at birth an individual's probability of developing a serious illness or disability over his or her lifetime, physicians can take immediate action to eliminate through genetic engineering or ameliorate through early intervention, thus saving hundreds of thousands, if not millions, of dollars in lifetime costs borne by payers and plans. Thus, not only does predict, prevent, and manage medicine potentially provide accurate comparable data for payers and plans to consider; it also comes with a potential set of solutions for dealing with the problems upstream in the value chain. If an intervention for a particular problem identified at birth does not currently exist, the advance knowledge nevertheless enables society to plan for handling the problem—for example, through the development of set-aside funds that could be allocated to plans and provider systems where these individuals enroll. But with the potential problem known at birth, there would also be an increased probability that an intervention might be developed (new drugs, for example, or biotech discoveries) to deal with it before the individual becomes a costly illness burden on the plan or provider system.

The second development relates to the increasing consolidation of both the insurer and provider components of the health care sector. The argument is frequently made that even with capitated payment, plans and providers have little incentive to engage in unusual acts of prevention or become involved in population-based community health improvement efforts because the plan or provider does not cover or provide for enough of the population to make it worthwhile. Further, given the mobility of the American population and the numbers of people who switch health plans each year, why should a health plan or provider system make an investment that may ultimately benefit its competitors? There is no financial return to the plan. In addition, mobility aside, the returns from such early prevention and health promotion efforts are largely long term and therefore are not likely to meet the short-run financial pressures facing the plan or delivery system.

But as health plans and providers consolidate, they begin to cover and provide care for ever-larger numbers of people. In California, the four largest health maintenance organizations (HMOs) account for 69 percent of the total HMO market (Schauffler and Brown, 1999). Integrated health plan and health provider systems such as the Henry Ford Health System in Detroit, Michigan, and Intermountain Health Care in Salt Lake City, Utah, bear responsibility for upward of 500,000 to 1 million lives and more. Although antitrust legislation and related concerns will place some limits on the ultimate degree of consolidation, we believe that consolidation on both the health plan and provider side will continue to be a growth business for many years. This expansion of the population base mitigates the argument of plans and providers that they have little economic incentive to make an investment in population-based health care improvement initiatives. First, with increased size, they can achieve greater economies of both scale and scope with their prevention and community health improvement efforts. Second, with increased size, they are not affected as much by the mobility of plan members or those who switch enrollment. Finally, with the increased size of the population covered and cared for, plans and providers have greater incentives and opportunities to realize the long-term gains of early investments.

Thus, we suggest that the current angst regarding continued cost-cutting efforts, restricted choice, great variations in service, technical quality, and outcomes of care associated with the ongoing march of managed care should be reframed as a search for value and new ways of creating value. We have suggested that value creation is shifting from investment in tangible assets of physical capital to the intangible assets of human capital, information, and knowledge capital and customer relationships. We have also suggested that the current primary emphasis on cost containment as a way of creating greater value will give way to a greater emphasis on quality and outcomes of care as we realize the huge value leakage resulting from unneeded costly variations in clinical practice and error rates and defects in treatment that would not be tolerated by most other sectors of the economy. We have further suggested that the new value frontier in the coming decades will be population-based health management, whereby plans and providers will be paid for keeping individuals and populations well. Advances in genetics and immunology and the growing consolidation of plans and providers themselves will reinforce this major transition. This will require a merger of medicine and management, public health and the community, some examples of which are discussed in subsequent chapters of this book. An additional major force for a value-driven health system, not merely a cost-driven health system, is the demand for new forms of accountability.

## Demand for Accountability

Four major factors influence the demand for new forms of accountability: (1) the resource-limiting incentives of managed care; (2) growing recognition of the wide variation in quality and outcomes of care, including evidence of errors that exceed those of most other sectors; (3) advances in the ability of health services research to measure quality and outcomes of care; and (4) the advance of information technology. Although there is no systematic scientific evidence to date that managed care's emphasis on cutting costs and incentives to constrain resource use has been associated with poorer quality or outcomes of care, there have been numerous media accounts of individuals and their families who have suffered or experienced poor outcomes of care allegedly due to the impositions of managed care. This led to the creation in 1998 of the President's Advisory Commission on Consumer Protection and Quality in the Health Care Industry, the demand for patient self-protection legislation at the federal and state levels, and the proposal for a national quality commission that would establish benchmark standards and monitor quality and outcomes of care. At least thirty-seven states publish some quality-of-care and outcome data (Millenson, 1997).

Aside from the concerns about managed care, there is also growing evidence that the quality and outcomes of care in the United States are not as good as we might have thought or hoped (Schuster, McGlynn, and Brook, 1998; Institute of Medicine, 2000b). There is widespread evidence of underuse of appropriate medical procedures, overuse of inappropriate and potentially harmful procedures, and misuse of appropriate procedures (Chassin, 1998; Chassin, Galvin, and the National Roundtable on Health Care Quality, 1998; Institute of Medicine, 2000b).

A related factor pushing for increased accountability is the advances made by health services researchers in developing more reliable and valid measures of quality and outcomes of care. Advances in risk-adjustment methodologies (Iezzoni, 1994) make it possible to compare outcomes for a number of conditions, including coronary artery bypass graft surgery, acute myocardial infarction, total hip replacement, and related procedures and conditions. New York, Pennsylvania, and California have published outcome data. The federal Agency for Health Care Policy and Research has also been an active funder, promoter, and disseminator of health care quality and outcomes data, including the funding and development of evidenced-based practice centers focusing on over twenty conditions and development of a national clearinghouse for clinical protocols and guidelines.

Finally, advances in information technology have enabled greater amounts of data to be processed faster and, through the Internet, shared with patients and the public at large. The result has been a feeding frenzy by the American public for health and medical data.

Taken as a whole, these factors have led to a transformation of health care accountability based on the trust inherent in the doctor-patient relationship to one based on data and evidence. In brief, we have moved from trust-based accountability to evidence-based accountability (Relman, 1988). This is reflected in the development of quality standards by the NCQA, the continued evolution of quality performance data by the JCAHCO, and the development of the American Medical Association's efforts to accredit physician groups based on quality criteria. At the same time, the number of stakeholders to whom physicians and health professionals are accountable has increased, frequently requiring the need to balance competing demands (Emanuel and Emanuel, 1996). Most significant, the four forces have led to a transfer of power among physicians, patients, and the public at large (Millenson, 1997). The result has been a democratization of the patient-physician relationship and the evolution of mutual accountability that extends beyond the medical profession to the involvement of payers, various accreditation bodies, and the public at large (Shortell, Waters, Clarke, and Budetti, 1998).

## Accountability: Individual and Community

The medical profession has long emphasized the individual clinical accountability of the physician for the health of the individual patient under the physician's care. Although this is obviously an important responsibility for which the profession will continue to be accountable, it is no longer sufficient. As providers assume more financial risk for maintaining and enhancing the health of their enrollees, responsibility and accountability for the health of larger aggregates of individuals are evolving (Kassirer, 1998). Physicians increasingly need to balance the allocation of limited resources between the immediate interest of individual patients and the potential future needs of other enrollees, as well as the financial risk to the physician and the practice organizations to which they belong. Increasingly physicians will need to take broader responsibility for the health of their enrolled population (Shortell, Waters, Clarke, and Budetti, 1998). Moreover, the profession will need to engage public health and community health organizations at large in dealing with such underlying problems as substance abuse, violence, teenage pregnancy, and involuntary injuries.

## Accountability: Paying for Population-Based Health Outcomes

As value is created for quality and outcome criteria in addition to cost criteria, payers will compensate providers for meeting the broader-based criteria. In the short run, this will be largely based on process quality criteria, such as the use of beta blockers at discharge for acute myocardial infarction patients, appropriate use of antibiotics for pneumonia, the use of warfarin for chronic atrial fibrillation, influenza immunization for the elderly, retinal eye exams and annual HbA1c hemoglobin testing for diabetes, mammography screening for breast cancer, and related process indicators. Over time, however, these indicators will evolve to more of an outcome orientation to reflect clinical markers and functional health status outcomes of people with acute myocardial infarction, congestive heart failure, stroke, diabetes, breast cancer, and so on (Siu and others, 1992).

Ultimately providers and payers alike will recognize the advantage of more "upstream" value creation that can be achieved through disease prevention and health promotion efforts to prevent acute myocardial infarction, congestive heart failure, stroke, diabetes, and related conditions from developing in the first place. Whether they do so will depend greatly on the extent to which providers are at financial risk for the health status of enrolled populations. For the age group below sixty-five years this will vary greatly across markets and states depending largely on private sector insurance and payment dynamics, but the Medicare program for those over age sixty-five will be a great leveler for everyone. Medicare (and, to a lesser extent, Medicaid) increasingly will hold providers financially accountable for the care rendered to recipients, and the number of at-risk contracts will continue to grow. Although these contracts may create incentives for earlier intervention and health-sustaining behaviors, the payments are still based on risk-adjusted predictions of the likely illness and disease burden of the population.

The breakthrough innovation in payment policy will be for the federal government or private payers to pay providers based on the health outcomes achieved (Kindig, 1997). An example of a global measure of outcomes is QALY, one way of achieving a measure of health-adjusted life expectancy (Williams, 1988, 1996; Gold, Franks, McCoy, and Fryback, 1998). Health-adjusted life expectancy calculations are based on a combination of length of life, disease, and disability. Financial incentives, such as bonuses and savings based on a reduction of work-loss days, will be provided to providers and plans showing the greatest improvement in the health status of the relevant populations over time. The purchase and payment of health care based on outcomes achieved will require not only well-integrated organized delivery systems across the medical–health care continuum but also cross-sector integration with public health, environment, housing, transportation, education, law enforcement, and social service sectors as well. In his pathbreaking book *Purchasing Population Health* (1997), Kindig outlines a three-phase program for achieving such a payment policy. Phase one, currently in process, involves further discussion and debate, advances in research, and selected demonstration projects. Phase two, roughly from the year 2000 to 2010, will involve an expansion of population-based outcome payment to integrated health care systems capable of assuming such responsibility. This would be followed by phase three (roughly 2011 to 2020), in which the environmental and social service sectors' contribution to population health would be incorporated. Although further advances are needed in population-based health needs assessment, health outcome measurement, standardization of information, and related factors, it is clear that paying for health produced rather than illness or disease treated is the gold standard in accountability from a value creation perspective. Although full-scale implementation may be years and even decades away, its logic is compelling.

2

# The Organized Delivery System
## *Ideal Versus Reality*

A n ideal health care system has the following characteristics:

- Focuses on meeting the health needs of individuals *and* populations

- Matches its resources, competencies, and capabilities to meet individual and population needs and objectives

- Involves patients in all aspects of their care

- Coordinates and integrates care across the continuum

- Develops a total and ongoing relationship with its patients

- Aims to provide a totally satisfying experience for the patient that embraces service quality as well as technical quality

- Guarantees that treatments known scientifically to be effective are given to patients who benefit from them (they avoid underuse), that treatments known to be harmful or of no use are not given to patients (they avoid overuse), and that knowledge about uncertain treatments continues to grow to reduce the uncertainty

- Has information systems to link patients, providers, and payers across the continuum of care

- Provides information on costs, quality, outcomes, and patient satisfaction to multiple stakeholders: patients, employees, staff, payers and purchasers, community groups, and external review bodies

- Uses financial incentives and organizational structure to align governance, management, physicians, and other caregivers in support of achieving shared objectives

- Is able to participate as an effective partner in the communitywide health care management system

- Is able to improve continuously the care that it provides

- Is able to learn and renew itself to continue to improve its work on all of the above elements

This book focuses on nine of the eleven organized delivery health care systems featured in the original edition. These nine systems were Advocate Health Care (Oak Brook, Illinois); Baylor Health Care System (Dallas, Texas); Fairview Health Services (Minneapolis, Minnesota); Franciscan Health System (Tacoma, Washington); Henry Ford Health System (Detroit, Michigan); Mercy Health Services (Farmington Hills, Michigan); Sentara Healthcare (Norfolk, Virginia), Sisters of Providence (Seattle, Washington); and Sutter Health (Sacramento, California). Sharp HealthCare (San Diego, California) and UniHealth (Burbank, California) did not participate in the update. In 1996 all of these systems were striving to become fully developed organized delivery systems (ODSs). One of the major objectives of this second edition was to reexamine where the systems stood four years later relative to their quest to become ODSs. A full discussion of the methods used in this update is in Resource A. As indicated in the Resource, part of this assessment included asking the members of the top management team of each system to evaluate their system on a scale of 1 to 5 in terms of eight elements reflecting some of the characteristics of an ideal health care system.

The results are shown in Table 2.1. A look at the average column shows that the systems rate themselves on the eight criteria in the range of 2.6 to 3.8. The highest average marks are given for the

Table 2.1. System Self-Assessment of
Ideal Elements in a Health Care System.

| Element | Average | Range |
| --- | --- | --- |
| 1  Focuses on meeting the population's health needs | 3.4 | 3.0–4.2 |
| 2  Matches services capacity to meet the populations' needs | 3.7 | 3.0–4.5 |
| 3  Coordinates and integrates care across the continuum | 3.5 | 3.0–4.0 |
| 4  Has information systems to link patients, providers, and payers across the continuum of care | 2.6 | 2.3–3.5 |
| 5  Is able to provide information on cost, quality outcomes, and patient satisfaction to multiple stakeholders: patients, staff, payers and purchasers, community groups, and external review bodies | 3.8 | 3.0–4.5 |
| 6  Uses financial incentives and organizational structure to align governance, management, physicians, and other caregivers in support of achieving shared objectives | 3.7 | 3.0–4.5 |
| 7  Is able to improve continuously the care that it provides | 3.3 | 2.0–4.7 |
| 8  Is willing and able to work with others to ensure that the community's health objectives are met | 3.8 | 3.5–5.0 |

Note: Averages are based on a minimum of four top management team respondents per system.

ability to provide information to multiple stakeholders and to being willing and able to work with others to meet community health objectives. The lowest grade is given in regard to having "information to link patients, providers and payers across the continuum of care." Only one system achieved an overall average grade of 4.0 across the eight elements. The remaining were in the 3.0 to 3.5 range. In brief, everyone acknowledges that they are far from where they want to be.

It is important to recognize that embedded within the ideal elements is a mix of health care delivery objectives and health objectives. The suggestion is that health care systems will need to be in both the health care delivery "business" and the health "business" if they are to play a viable role in their communities and with the American public at large. Clearly this goal will require a new vision, an expanded set of competencies and capabilities, a new understanding of how value is created, a redeployment of capital and other assets, and the willingness to work with new partners. To restore, maintain, and enhance health will require a new vehicle, of which the organized health care delivery system will be a part. We call this vehicle the community health care management system and develop its key features in Chapter Seven. This chapter reviews the evidence on the performance of organized delivery systems (ODSs).

## Have Organized Delivery Systems Achieved Value?

In the first edition of this book, we suggested that remaking health care in America would need to be centered around developing more organized systems of care that reduce fragmentation and redundancy and promote greater continuity of care, thus enhancing quality and outcomes using as few necessary resources as possible. We also suggested that such systems of care would be particularly important for managing chronic illness, which frequently cuts across specialized expertise and involves the coordination of multiple providers. We went on to suggest that organized delivery systems would enjoy a comparative advantage to the extent that payment for services would become increasingly capitated. Although we were not able to measure quality or outcomes of care, we did find some evidence that the organized delivery systems we were studying that were more integrated did experience a lower increase in costs (Shortell, Gillies, and Anderson, 1994). We also found that greater standardization of key support functions—human resources, strategic planning, information systems, and quality assurance—was positively associated with a greater degree of physician integration and clinical integration. Most elements of physician integration were in turn positively associated with greater total system revenue and cash flow. Physician integration was also strongly associated with clinical integration. Despite these associations, we observed that the absolute levels of both perceived and objective measures of integration were relatively modest on most dimensions and that significant internal and external barriers to achieving more integrated systems of care were identified. Not the least among these was a payment environment that, if anything, promoted conflicting financial incentives and continued fragmentation of service delivery.

What has happened over the past four years? First, the growth of capitated payment has slowed, and a mix of payment arrangements continues to exist. This produces conflicting incentives for providers, for example, increasing hospitalization under per case reimbursement versus reducing hospitalization under global capitation arrangements. In brief, aligned financial incentives to provide more coordinated integrated care do not exist.

Second, most of the integration efforts of health systems have been overly focused on cost reductions rather than on overall value improvement and seeking additional revenue opportunities. As Drucker (1998) notes, "The HMO has been attempting to base the integration of health care management on costs—that is, managing the system to minimize its costs rather than to maximize health care. To be successfully integrated, the management of health care delivery will surely have to be based on health care rather than on finance" (p. 172).

Third, the challenge of clinical integration has proved tougher than most predicted. Not the least of the challenge is the fact that most physicians still practice in solo or very small partnerships and groups, making it extremely difficult to link them to serious efforts to integrate patient care across the continuum. The clinical integration challenge has been compounded by the disparate cultures and incentives associated with managing hospitals, physician groups, and insurance plans. In addition, the high cost of implementing computerized patient records and developing integrated clinical and financial information systems has been a major barrier.

Fourth has been an unfortunate misunderstanding on the part of the press, other media, and other observers who have largely interpreted an integrated delivery system in terms of owned vertical integration, that is, a system having direct ownership of the different stages of the production process, such as hospitals, physician groups, nursing homes, and so on. As a result, any actions taken by such systems to move out of direct ownership of health plans, physician groups, or related arrangements to contractual relationships for such services has been viewed as "dis-integration" (Advisory Board, 1997) and cited as a failure of integrated health systems. These observers apparently do not allow for virtual integration mechanisms built around contractual relationships and strategic alliances, which frequently can offer more flexibility and potentially lower costs. Most organized delivery systems today in fact are hybrid organizations, containing both owned and nonowned components. The issue of ownership versus contractual alliance is a major issue in all sectors and has been greatly influenced by transaction costs economics arguments (Williamson, 1975, 1981, 1985; Robinson, 1997; Conrad and Shortell, 1996).

Finally, integrated and organized delivery systems have been criticized on the ground that they are too large and bureaucratic and unable to meet emerging customer demands (Herzlinger, 1996).

These critics put forward "focused factories" as the answer to our health care problems. Focused factories are based, in part, on Fredrick Taylor's principles of scientific management first developed in 1911 (Taylor, 1947). The idea is to match professional expertise to the job, focusing on specific conditions or illnesses and relying on volume and learning curve effects to achieve superior outcomes at lower costs. Carve-out heart hospitals, cancer centers, and single-illness disease management companies serve as examples. Although value can be created by focusing expertise and resources on given conditions, the focused factory approach looks backward to the health system of the 1950s to the 1980s, which was characterized by a high volume of acute care delivered largely in hospitals. It is unlikely to be a viable model for dealing with the multiple chronic illnesses that Americans now face. How is a diabetic heart patient with asthma, for example, served by a focused factory? How are the needs of a mother with breast cancer who cares for a mother-in-law with chronic obstructive pulmonary disease and has a child at home with attention deficit disorder served by a focused factory? How do focused factories deal with teenage pregnancy, substance abuse, and domestic violence? A focused factory approach can achieve some success with limited conditions, but the danger is that focused factories will create even larger silos than the ones that many organized delivery systems are trying to eliminate.

## Evidence on the Performance of Organized Delivery Systems

Approximately 72 percent of U.S. hospitals belong to a network (assets are not owned) or system (based on asset ownership): 2,467 hospitals belong to 306 networks, and 3,017 hospitals belong to 297 systems (Bazzoli and others, 1999). Since 1996, relatively little systematic empirical work on the performance of organized delivery systems or networks has occurred, and the evidence that does exist is largely mixed (Snail and Robinson, 1998). Some find that systems organized primarily around vertically integrated owned facilities experience poorer performance (Walston and Bogue, 1999; Walston, Kimberly, and Burns, 1996). This may be due to diseconomies of scale created by systems that have grown too large (Robinson and Casalino, 1996). Internal transfer pricing problems may also arise in regard to hospital, physician group, and health plan relationships when all three entities are owned (Burns and Thorpe, forthcoming). Ownership of all components may also raise issues of where and with whom to fix accountability. On the other hand, in comparison with totally independent hospitals, system hospitals have lower average costs and marginal costs (Menke, 1997; Snail and Robinson, 1998).

In the area of hospital-physician integration, the evidence is also mixed (Dynan, Bazzoli, and Burns, 1998). Some have found tighter forms of integration (salary and equity models) to be associated with either higher costs or no impact at all on costs (Alexander and Morrisey, 1988; Goes and Zhan, 1995; Conrad and others, 1996). Hospitals that have purchased primary care practices have consistently lost money (Burns, Cacciamani, Clement, and Aquino, 2000; Hill and Wild, 1995). Most recently, Snail (1999) found an association between hospital-physician integration and higher costs except for hospital contracting with group practices. It is important to note that much of the literature is limited by a lack of relevant available data as well as the inability to take into account selection bias in the samples studied.

A recent study based on national data found that systems with asset-based ownership of most of its components exhibited superior financial performance on multiple dimensions than the more loosely organized networks (Bazzoli, Chan, and Shortell, 1999). Consistent with Williamson (1981, 1985) and others (Conrad and Shortell, 1996), ownership may reduce the transaction costs associated with monitoring contractual relationships and alliances. Ownership may also result in quicker, more focused decision making than can be achieved with the more loosely organized networks in which individual hospitals typically retain policymaking authority. Interest-

ingly, more centralized networks achieve greater financial performance than less centralized networks do, and a curvilinear relationship between centralization and financial performance existed
for systems (Bazzoli, Chan, and Shortell, 1999). Systems that were
moderately centralized outperformed those that were either highly
centralized or decentralized. The issue appears to be one of balancing the economies of scale and scope that can be achieved with
increasing size and centralization with the need to stay in touch
with local markets and fast-changing environments (Robinson,
1997, 1999b). The proper mix of ownership and centralization of
relationships depends on local market dynamics and history, the
internal capabilities of the system, and the current and future capabilities of potential alliance partners. As others have concluded in
studying sectors outside health care, "If firms lack the internal
mechanisms needed to exploit the advantages integration can provide—if they lack the bargaining power to win concessions from
suppliers (or from distributors or customers), or if their industries
become highly volatile—then the strategic outlet for vertical integration does not look good" (Harrigan, 1980, p. 424).

Some observers have suggested that more highly integrated
delivery systems are better able to generate the levels of quality and
outcome data demanded by NCQA and related groups (Zelman,
1996). Such systems are more likely to have the resources to invest
in information systems and related infrastructure needed for Continuous Quality Improvement (CQI). In contrast, more loosely
organized systems built on contractual relationships and strategic
alliances may offer greater flexibility in regard to costs of production and pricing (Zelman, 1996).

But Bazzoli, Chan, and Shortell (1999) found that more centralized systems and networks enjoyed greater financial performance
than systems and networks composed largely of autonomous hospitals, physician organizations, and health plans.

The evidence on integration of services outside the acute care
sector is largely positive. For example, Rosenheck, Frisman, and

Kasparow (1999) found that the integration of Veterans Administration clinical staff time with that of social security personnel significantly improved access to disability benefits for homeless veterans. Others have found that services for people with mental illness are more effective when delivered in integrated systems (Rosenheck and others, 1998; Lehman and others, 1994; Beiser, Shore, Peters, and Tatum, 1985).

Thus, the relatively sparse empirical evidence to date suggests that the ability of organized delivery systems to add value, particularly within the larger context of community- and population-based health improvement, may depend more on certain core competencies and capabilities than on ownership models. Building on the foundation of our earlier work and the value creation chains shown in Figure 1.1, we suggest three capabilities (Gillies and others, 1993):

> *Functional integration*—the extent to which key support functions and activities (such as financial management, strategic planning, human resource management, and information management) are coordinated across operating units so as to add the greatest overall value to the systems

> *Physician integration*—the extent to which physicians are economically linked to a system, use its facilities and services, and actively participate in its planning, management, and governance

> *Clinical integration*—the extent to which services are coordinated across people, functions, activities, and sites over time to as to maximize the value of care delivered to patients

The most important of the functional integration capabilities are those associated with the deployment of human resource strategies, information technology, and continuous improvement processes. The most important of the physician integration capabilities are those associated with the development of true physician groups and a depth of leadership that can help build trusting relationships. And the most important capability associated with clinical integration is the implementation of care management systems across the continuum of care that also link with community health care management issues in such a way as to track outcomes of health improvement efforts for individual patients and the community at large over time.

In the following chapters, we examine the progress that our original study systems have made in developing these capabilities, examine their governance and management systems, and assess the future prospects for integrated health care as a foundation for the development of community health care management systems.

# 3

# Functional Integration

Functional integration is defined as the extent to which key support functions and activities (such as financial management, human resources, strategic planning, information management, marketing, and quality improvement) are coordinated across operating units so as to add the greatest overall value to the system. In the most general sense, integration involves shared or common policies and practices for each of these functions. However, high centralization and standardization do not automatically translate into a high level of integration. The degree of integration depends on what the consequences of centralization and standardization are. What distinguishes the integration of a function or service is that the function or service serves all the components of the system in a coordinated manner and adds value to the system overall. The good of the system is paramount.

The purpose behind the integration of human resource functions, for example, is not merely the establishment of common policies and processes but rather the establishment of policies and processes that facilitate the movement of resources within and between operating units to where they are needed at any particular time. The more the human resource functions of a system allow the system to use its human resources to its best advantage, the more functionally integrated the human resource policies and processes are. Financial management processes are more integrated the more they allow budgeting and capital allocation that emphasize the needs of the system overall instead of individual operating unit goals. Integrated financial management functions enable the system to shift resources around the system so as to maximize the system's capacity. The more the strategic plans of the various units in the system are based on a set of common guidelines and goals that are designed to improve the system, the higher the degree of integration there is. Integration of information systems occurs when there is an exchange of data within and among a system's operating units that promotes cost-effective care across the continuum and overall clinical and fiscal responsibility. Quality improvement efforts are more integrated the more they are common or shared throughout the system and promote the mutual learning required for the continuous improvement of quality.

It is important to note, however, that not all functional and service areas need to be or should be integrated for physician and clinical integration to advance and for the system to improve its performance. Some areas may be more important to integrate than others may. Williams (1992) noted that centralization and standardization made sense only when they would result in significant economies of scale or improved expertise. He viewed CQI and TQM planning, budgeting, information, and communication as areas that were likely to be especially good candidates. But there is no firm rule regarding any of these or others. The functions and services that should be integrated are somewhat idiosyncratic to each system due to such factors as the environment it faces and its structural arrangement.

In our earlier work, we reported results from self-administered structured (closed-ended) questionnaires that surveyed system-level and operating unit–level management regarding their perceptions of various aspects (functional, physician-system, and clinical) of their system's integration in 1991 and 1992. These results indicated that the systems had achieved at best a moderate level of overall functional integration, with a score of 3.0 on a 1 (low) to 5 (high) scale in both years. Of the nine specific functional areas covered in the surveys, the areas that participants indicated the greatest integration were financial management (operating policies and resource allocation), culture, and strategic planning, with scores ranging between 3.1 and 3.4. Human resources and quality assurance were in the midrange. Information services, support services, and marketing were the least integrated, with scores between 2.5 and 2.7. There was relatively little change during the time of the study. This is the case even for the two functional areas, information services and quality assurance, which were assessed again in 1994. Analyses in the earlier work demonstrated some statistical support for the relationships between the factors hypothesized to be associated with functional integration and between functional integration and physician integration and clinical integration. However, the strength of these relationships was not as strong as one might hope, a fact that could perhaps be attributed to the relatively early stages of the integration process at the time. The patterns were not yet clearly established or observable.

## Recent Update

In the earlier study, many systems were uncertain about which functional areas were most important to integrate and thus undertook the integration of most of their functions and services. But as many of these efforts met with failure or problems, system leaders began to target specific functions and services that made sense in their situation. Between the time of the original study and this follow-up, many systems found by trial and error that in their circumstances, certain functions or services should or could be integrated and others should not or could not be integrated.

Key system leaders were surveyed in the summer of 1999 regarding the status of functional, physician, and clinical integration efforts at their systems. (Resource A provides details on the data collection process.) These system leaders were asked to assess how important the integration of each of a number of functions, services, and elements was for the system's plans. The results of the survey indicate that financial management and operating policies and information systems were considered most important to integrate, with scores of 3.0 on the 1 (not very important) to 3 (very important) scale. Financial management and resource allocation, quality assurance and quality improvement, and strategic planning were also viewed as very important (all had average scores of 2.9) areas to integrate for the success of the system, with the least important being administrative support (2.3). Of somewhat less importance were human resources (2.7) and marketing (2.7).

The results of the 1999 surveys show that most of the systems have located these functions primarily at the system level, with occasional sharing of power with the operating unit or regional unit. Several health care systems locate these functions primarily at the regional level. Respondents are most satisfied with their progress on strategic planning and financial management and operating policies (each with an average score of 3.8 on a scale of 1, for the lowest satisfaction, to 5, for the highest satisfaction) and least satisfied with information systems (average score of 2.7). This low score for information systems is especially interesting given its perceived importance for physician and clinical integration and overall system integration. The integration efforts for many of these functions, services, and elements, including those for administrative support, financial management, and strategic planning, have been usually within one to twelve months of being on schedule. However, the system leaders indicated that in other areas, most notably information systems and quality assurance and quality improvement efforts, their systems were over a year behind schedule. Some attributed the tardiness of their effort to focusing on year 2000 (Y2K) computer issues. But some also noted that the delay caused by this focus on Y2K issues actually may benefit them. During the delay, Internet technology and capabilities developed so much that it may be a major component of the solution to their information system inte-

gration problems. Quality assurance and quality improvement delays were often attributed to system emphasis on cost issues rather
than quality issues and on the lack of progress on infofmation systems. The emphasis on cost saving was also seen as one of the major
reasons that system efforts to promote a shared culture were behind
schedule.

## Barriers and Challenges to Integration

In our earlier work, we identified a number of barriers to the attempts of systems to achieve integration. Based on telephone interviews with key system leaders at the nine systems featured here
(see Resource A), one of these barriers has become less important.
The lack of geographic concentration of operating units is no longer
a significant problem; systems seem to have rationalized their
makeup by unbundling operating units that did not help create a
coherent whole. But a number of previously identified obstacles,
sometimes in modified form, as well as a new one exist: lack of operating unit commitment to the integration strategy, continued
focus on the operating unit, diversions of merger activity, lack of
understanding of integration, inability to identify the key functions
to integrate, lack of trained personnel, and inadequate information
systems.

### Lack of Operating Unit Commitment to Integration

The unwillingness of some of the system's operating units to join in
the system's integration efforts continues to be a barrier for many
systems. A number of systems still confront operating units that
fight to maintain their autonomy. The operating units of some systems, especially hospitals, continue to enjoy positive bottom lines
and thus have not felt the need to buy into the system strategy of
integration. The system may allow a financially successful operating unit to proceed with its own plans as long as it has the ability
to fund them. Or a financially successful operating unit may be

allowed to lead the entire system in a direction that benefits itself more than the system overall. The more successful units often do not want to integrate financial functions because they do not want to give up their control of revenues and share their bounty with other components of the system. In addition, in a number of systems, many of the operating units are reluctant to support system integration activities financially. In general, there is often little willingness to sacrifice individual operating units for the good of the system or to see how helping others in the system actually benefits all of the system's components.

### Continued Focus on the Operating Unit

Integration is also inhibited by the inability of a system to change its focus as well as the focus of its individual operating units to the system overall. In 1996 we described this as a hospital focus. This must be broadened somewhat given the extent to which systems now include health plan or physician group components. At the individual level, this operating unit focus means that many of the individuals in the system continue to identify with and owe their allegiances to the individual operating unit. As a result, efforts to integrate various functions are hindered because operating unit–oriented employees consider the needs of the system as secondary to those of the operating unit. For example, integrated human resource policies may require employees with enough flexibility to work at whichever system site has needs at a particular time; operating unit–oriented people may not be able or willing to do this.

At the operating unit level, this barrier is manifested by the continued focus on the individual component part of the system rather than the system as a whole. One of the most problematic examples is that although the goal is system integration and the good of the system overall, performance of the system is often evaluated in terms of its components parts, not of the system overall. It is not uncommon for operating units performing less well to complain that their lesser performance is due to accounting procedures, that is, a shifting of costs and revenues, that hurt them and help another unit. This is a frequent complaint of physician groups that system accounting often shows to be in the red. The members of the physician groups maintain that the group is not being given credit for the revenues it brings in downstream. Nor do they receive credit for revenues such as ancillary services that the physicians used to enjoy but were reallocated to the system when the physicians became part of a system-affiliated group. These revenues become part of a hospital's positive bottom line while the physician group shows a negative bottom line. Such operating units argue that the unit comparisons are contrary to the system orientation that the integration effort is supposed to be promoting.

### Diversions of Merger Activity

The leaders of a number of systems have seen mergers as offering great opportunities for their systems to improve their market position and build a coherent system. However, in the process of trying to improve the system through merger, many of these systems have experienced reversals or delays of their integration activities, regardless of whether these mergers are successfully completed. Two primary factors cause the reversals or delays. First, huge amounts of staff and resources are diverted from integration-related activities to merger-related activities. Second, staff and resources not devoted to merger activities often are not put to work on integration efforts because of the uncertainty of whether any work accomplished will survive the merger. The result of the diversion of and reluctance to commit staff and resources is that integration activity often comes to a standstill during merger talks. Even if merger efforts are successful and the health care systems do join together, the merger may cause even more problems as the new organization tries to meld the two former systems together into a coherent new whole. The more dissimilar the members of the new health care system are, the more effort must be expended in creating a coherent whole from the component parts. Much merger activity has occurred throughout the country and among the study systems since 1996. Fairview Health Services/University of Minnesota Hospital, Sentara Healthcare/Tidewater Health System, and Baylor Health Care System/Texas Health Resources are just a few of the examples of merger activities, both successful and unsuccessful, that the systems in the study have experienced. Each of these efforts had some negative impact on the system's integration efforts.

## Lack of Understanding of Integration

In many systems, there is a lack of understanding as to what integration means—system, functional, physician-system, or clinical. This is less of an obstacle than in the past because the leaders of most systems have made a concerted effort to provide some definition to the concept. But there is still no fully integrated health care system to serve as a model to which leaders can point as an example of their goal or demonstrate the benefits that they seek to achieve. Some operating unit personnel still perceive system attempts at integration as merely a corporate attempt to usurp power. System leaders still struggle to implement a design of the organized delivery system.

## Inability to Identify Key Functions to Integrate

Many systems are still trying to determine which functions should be integrated, that is, which better serve the system standardized or centralized and which are more beneficial if not. The answer to these questions is in part dependent on external factors, such as the market environment. It is also dependent on what a modern health system's core business is. The new core business for many health care systems continues to shift from acute inpatient care to primary care, wellness, and the continuum of care. The need to integrate functions must be judged on the basis of the impact of such an action on the creation of a seamless continuum of care and what is best for the patient, not on financial economies of scale or scope alone.

### Lack of Trained Personnel

Problems with personnel relate not only to shifts from site to site but also shifts from function to function. Clinically, care for the patient across the continuum requires a vast array of expertise in a number of settings. Advances in technology have changed the requirements of many jobs in the health care system. In addition, continuity of care argues for patient contact with fewer people who have more skills. However, a number of factors prevent systems from using system personnel to either the system's or the patient's best advantage. Most systems confront state and federal limitations (such as licensing requirements and regulations) on the use of their personnel and also face union limitations. Even if these factors are overcome, in many cases personnel with the necessary skills (either specialized skills or multiple skills) are not available. Many systems also have suffered from a high turnover in management, especially at the middle level. The Balanced Budget Act of 1997 required substantial cutbacks at all clinical and managerial levels of many systems, resulting in high levels of insecurity for many. One leader described resulting middle management behavior as "Machiavellian." At both the managerial and the clinical levels, systems are often trying to perform "new (health care) world" tasks using personnel in "old (health care) world" positions with "old world" skills. Efforts to integrate the human resource function or the support services function are often thwarted.

### Inadequate Information Systems

Information systems continue to be a major impediment to integration for all of the systems examined. In spite of millions, if not billions, of dollars spent on information systems, none of the information systems of these health care systems is sufficiently developed to where it is a true asset for physician and clinical integration. This is because most of this money was spent on Y2K issues. The continued lack of agreement about what the information system should be like inhibits system integration. Most of the study systems would characterize their information systems as inadequate for their integration efforts. None of the participating systems has an information system that can link all the key actors (for example, primary care physician, hospital, home care) involved in the typical episode of care for a patient or allow the system to determine costs and outcomes of treatments effectively. Nor do most systems have a common patient identifier that allows such information to be linked among sites.

A few systems are relatively far along in assembling the pieces of an information system, but none has implemented a full-scale system. Agreement as to what the components of such a system should be, what information must be shared, and what does not have to be shared is slowly developing. Some systems have been able to implement either common financial information systems or at least one that allows for some compatibility with other operating units. Most operating units do have a clinical information system, limited as it may be, and are working toward systemwide standards that would allow cross-unit comparisons and exchange of data, as well as the merging of financial data with clinical data to enable cost-effectiveness and cost-benefit analyses.

## Key Success Factors and Some Best Practices

In spite of the barriers to integration, a number of the systems have been able to increase not only the level of integration of specific functions but also overall integration. These systems have used a variety of mechanisms and approaches, no single one of which would be adequate and not all of which would be suitable in all situations. However, a number of key success factors for functional integration specifically and integration overall can be identified. Although these factors are discussed separately, they are often interrelated and work together to promote integration.

### Strategic Plan

Key to integration is the development of a strategic plan that details a system's vision and goals and how the system intends to achieve them. Ideally, the plan should be based on a health status needs assessment of a population or community. The strategic plan should link short-run issues to long-run goals, the little picture to the big picture. An organized delivery system must act in terms of its strategic plans and long-range goals, with the caveat that these plans and goals must be flexible enough to change with the changing needs of the population. For example, acquisition, merger, and affiliation efforts must be evaluated much more strategically in order to increase the likelihood that the system has the right pieces in the right places. A successful organized delivery system will evaluate all opportunities in relation to its population-based strategic plans and long-range goals: Is this acquisition, merger, or affiliation necessary to meet the needs of the population it serves? Does this move contribute to system integration efforts? In addition, system leaders need to ensure that the system is strategically aligned: Are management control systems matched with market strategy? Are incentives aligned with strategy? Are resources aligned with strategy? Proposed new services should be evaluated in terms of the system strategy.

As a number of the system leaders interviewed suggested, providing a clear strategic plan that lays out the course for all members of the system is critical to obtaining the buy-in and compliance of those system members. Most of the leaders suggested that the strategic plan must have at least a three-year time frame in order to give system members time to implement it. In addition, the strategic plan should include methods and measures by which system and operating unit progress on that strategic plan can be assessed.

Most of the systems in the study are paying increased attention to alignment of strategy and actions. In the early 1990s the Baylor Health Care System did little formal strategic planning. However, in 1994 Baylor identified strategic planning as one of the key seven core processes that it needed to develop in order to work toward becoming a fully integrated health care system. As a result of a reengineering effort, Baylor now has a systemwide strategic plan that provides direction for the system as well as ways to assess its progress on that journey. Fairview, Henry Ford, and Mercy, among others, explicitly incorporate population-based planning and community health status needs in their strategic plans. Sentara developed a five-year strategic plan that is updated and evaluated annually. Management, board, and physicians were involved in its development. In addition to the overall system goals and plans included in the strategic plan, Sentara also developed subgoals and action plans that tie the activity of the system's operating units to the overall plan.

## Leadership

Strong system leadership committed to the integration process is instrumental. System leaders must communicate the vision, strategy, and understanding of system integration throughout the system. Members of a system need to understand what system leaders mean by "system integration" and its component parts: functional, physician-system, and clinical integration. Increased understanding of integration should reduce fears and beliefs that integration must surely adversely affect not only the individual (as with downsizing) but also the operating unit with which the individual identifies. Leaders need to emphasize the positive outcomes for patients, employees, operating units, and the system. And if the argument for system integration is going to be accepted by both administrative and clinical components of the system, the argument must go beyond cost and efficiency to include issues regarding patient care and quality.

Three of the systems have undergone top leadership change. What has remained constant, however, is the commitment of the top leadership to the notion of system integration. All still believe that the best model for their system to pursue its mission and vision is the integrated delivery system model. The system leaders at each of the various study systems have made and continue to make concerted efforts to communicate to employees, boards, and affiliated personnel information concerning system culture, system goals, and the integration effort. All of the systems employ a variety of techniques, including newsletters, retreats, telephone conferencing and videoconferencing, and face-to-face meetings as communication vehicles. For most, this intrasystem communication is a priority. For example, the CEO of Sutter Health decided to accept only two outside speaking engagements each year. He spends much of his time visiting the operating units that make up Sutter Health, interacting with the members of these operating units firsthand.

### Operating Unit Buy-In

Gaining the operating units' buy-in of integration plans is crucial for success, and key to this is bringing the operating unit leaders on board. Much attention must be given to these managers and associated implementation issues because they often do not see a need to change as quickly as system executives want. As a result, they can derail any integration efforts.

There are a number of approaches to achieving operating unit buy-in, or at least reducing the insular orientation of a system's operating units. First, clear communication of the strategic role each operating unit is to play in the overall system and regional strategy can help alleviate operating unit concerns. In addition, the system needs to find ways to change the focus of the operating unit leaders from their own hospital to the system as a whole. Advocate Health Care, Fairview, and Franciscan Health System gave their hospital leaders cross-system management responsibilities. The system can put chairs of the individual hospital boards on the overall system board and can create an office of governance for supporting all operating entity and systemwide governance activities. Sentara consolidated its governance boards into one. Many of these approaches are described in Chapter Six.

### Culture

A strong system culture is important to the integration process. To become more functionally integrated, the system must develop ways to get beyond the unit-based orientation of many of those working within the system. This is not to say that individual unit variation cannot be allowed within the system. However, the overarching values should be those of the system, and primary allegiance should be to the system. Systems need to develop a strong culture (at least in terms of the core values) that will promote a system perspective and provide a platform for additional integration work. Williams (1992) views "management culture [as] one of the most powerful tools to promote integration" (pp. 43–44). Although recognizing that changing a system's culture is difficult and time-consuming, Williams suggests that system leaders should "assess and monitor your culture [and] focus culture changes on the areas that will truly further integration" (p. 44), which include decision making, organizational integration, management style, management compensation, and management development. Building a common culture has become especially problematic given the number of mergers and affiliations that many health care systems have experienced.

A potentially very effective approach to building a common culture is through the implementation of CQI as the operating principles of the organization. A number of other means to enhance cultural values can be identified. By incorporating its mission, values, and philosophy (MVP) into its strategic plan, Advocate Health Care furthers the development of culture. The Advocate 2000 initiative helps promote the system's culture by development of associates' (employee and affiliated members of its health care community) understanding of how to integrate faith-based values better in their daily work lives. Linking performance appraisal and compensation incentives to expression of the system's cultural values and to managerial behavior consistent with those values has helped promote the development of Franciscan's culture. Defining itself as a "values-driven" organization, Sentara annually evaluates how successful the system has been in fulfilling its values, thus making the shared vision a priority for many.

A number of other mechanisms can be effective in developing a common culture and system orientation. Some systems use special ceremonies and celebrations to reinforce system values and culture. For example, Sentara has semiannual management meetings and CQI celebrations, and it has developed employee orientation videos that emphasize its culture and values. Fairview has used value clarification processes by which the system values are communicated throughout the system. The use of cross-unit task forces can also help facilitate joint programmatic efforts and get the members of a system more comfortable working with each other. Systems can institute joint programmatic planning and technology assessment planning across operating units. Cross-unit quality improvement activities are also used to help integrate various functional activities. Mercy Health Services uses such interunit teams and task forces in many of its efforts. They serve not only to build a stronger common culture but also help spread the learning throughout the system.

Systems should explore all opportunities to integrate, including initiating or expanding shared or common dietary, maintenance, housekeeping, security, and other support systems systemwide. Sentara has developed cross-unit support services. Advocate's reassigning personnel to new operating units helped to break down barriers between the two organizations that merged to form Advocate and to create a strong common culture in a relatively short period of time. In addition, system councils, meetings, and task forces that cut across all operating entities in functional areas such as nursing, human resources, marketing, and planning can be established to encourage input on a systemwide basis. Advocate Health Care and Henry Ford are among the study systems that have employed such systemwide groups. Fairview created functional integration teams that work on consolidation and standardization of services across the system.

Several systems are exploring the use of a shared service model to help facilitate functional integration and a common culture. For example, Henry Ford's model is characterized by having an operating unit's CEO retain operational control for a function or service, such as purchasing or human resources, but the function or service is centralized from a staff perspective in order to gain economies of scale and scope. Mercy Health Services' new shared services structure has moved such services as human resources, financial management, and materials management from the corporate office to the regional level. A team of corporate office and field people plus two CEO champions developed the plan for which functions should be located where. There are now three such regional centers in Michigan.

## Continuous Quality Improvement and Total Quality Management

Quality improvement activities, especially those using CQI/TQM approaches, can be beneficial for integration efforts for several reasons. First, CQI/TQM is itself a management philosophy and approach that, if adopted by a system, helps define a common view of the world and thus a common culture. A CQI culture can provide the key ingredient "needed to run health care systems thoughtfully, efficiently, and safely" (Goldsmith, 1998b, p. 76). Second, the techniques of CQI/TQM tend to promote systems thinking by focusing on the linkages of processes and activities across functions and units. Finally, CQI/TQM projects often require personnel in different units or functional areas to work together. These CQI/TQM activities must be linked explicitly to the system's strategic priorities so that they contribute to the integration process of the system.

Most of the study systems use CQI/TQM as a means to strengthen cultural values and develop an overall sense of systemness. For example, most of the systems use cross-unit meetings, councils, teams, or task forces in their CQI/TQM efforts, thus building bridges among their operating units and groups. Mercy has made this cross-unit team approach a cornerstone of its efforts to integrate and improve. It is committed to developing an "intelligent network" to promote the sharing of learning across the system. The system sponsors conferences and meetings that bring together representatives from its component units, thus building a common Mercy identity. Advocate and Sutter use the CQI process to build system identity in the lower levels of their system by involving coworkers in the selection of recipients of awards. Advocate and Henry Ford have used "system universities" that teach CQI methods to promote the values and culture of the system. Ford also has a board-level quality committee that is actively involved in the systems quality efforts. This committee attends Ford's annual Health Quality Fair at which fifty to sixty teams make presentations on various projects. This board involvement helps maintain system focus on quality.

## Information Systems

An integrated information system is both a key factor in the development of an organized delivery system and a consequence of that development: improving information systems helps system integration, and system integration helps develop information systems. Continued emphasis should be placed on developing clinical and management information systems as a foundation for facilitating overall integration efforts. However, information system development must be linked to the system's vision and strategic plan. The information needs of the various customers (community, patients, caregivers, payers, external accountability groups) must be defined. The information systems of an organized delivery system should be designed around these needs and incorporate relational data that can link patients and providers across the continuum. Information system integration efforts should focus on information that can be used for continuous improvement.

Although information system deficiencies should not be used as an excuse to avoid integration initiatives, information systems are nonetheless a key factor in achieving integration objectives. Recognizing this, many of the study's systems as well as other systems throughout the country are investing heavily in their information systems. To this point, much of this investment has gone to resolving Y2K issues. But more and more efforts are beginning to shift to developing information systems that add value to the integration of the system and provision of better care of the individuals served.

As is the case with many other systems, Advocate's approach to information systems development is to have a centralized information technology budget but also to incorporate some flexibility by allowing individual operating units to supplement the centralized budget with their own funds. These supplemental funds are typically used to provide for unit-based support personnel. One system has developed a patient registry that provides the primary care physicians with automated information on patients within the system (Arthur Andersen and American Hospital Association, 1999b). Physicians are able to identify which of their patients have certain diseases or conditions, are overdue for exams, or have problematic test results. Another system has developed a system to track patient satisfaction scores and allow comparison at the system, regional, clinic, and individual physician levels. Examples from outside the study systems include Intermountain Health Care, which has developed the Quality Care Tracking System that enables it to track clinical process improvements and link these improvements with system goals. Virginia Mason Medical Center (VMMC) has implemented an information system that can be accessed from anywhere within the Virginia Mason system. It uses Enterprise Wide Solutions, an information system with an outpatient care focus. VMMC has about 286 applications functioning. Data sets are automated and integrated across the system and include inpatient and outpatient records and scheduling. Although there are still issues of system reliability and full functionality, the general response has been positive.

In addition to spending about $50 million on Y2K conversion, Henry Ford has had some success in implementing its clinical information systems. The system has six clinics with computerized patient records that are totally paperless and plans to have all of its clinics paperless by the end of 2000. Henry Ford has an electronic reminder system for the approximately twenty-four thousand diabetic patients that the system serves. Ford is in the process of disseminating Care Plus, an intranet application to assist providers in delivering care by providing information on patient outcomes and guidelines for patient management. Ford's investment in IT is now proceeding more slowly due to financial reversals and examination of whether to outsource some of information technology efforts. But system leaders nevertheless believe that these efforts have been helpful in moving their integration efforts forward.

Sentara has seen information technology as critical to its integration efforts. All of its units are on the same general accounting system, which has produced standardization on a number of functions and services. All facilities use an identical chart form for accounts. Four of Sentara's six hospitals use the same set of clinical systems, including the lab system, patient scheduling, and the standard desktop. The Sentara physician information network is a Web-based physician communication mechanism by which physicians can examine histories and reports via the system's intranet. Sentara is working toward a system information system that can be used dynamically in all facets of managing a patient's care. The standardization of systems facilitates Sentara's ability to move personnel from one site to another because processes are identical in different operating units.

## Systemwide Incentives for Individuals

Individual performance appraisal systems that emphasize cooperative interdependent work can be used to promote cross-system integration. Compensation and incentives should be aligned to reinforce cross-system and cross-functional integration achievements; performance appraisal and compensation incentives should be linked to expression of the system's cultural values and systemwide strategies and to managerial behavior consistent with those values

and strategies. Study systems are now typically basing some of incentive pay for system executives on system performance levels.
Fairview executives have 20 percent of their pay at risk, with 60
percent of that being based on systemwide performance. Sutter
Health has established five-year financial targets with common incentives for managers. The top managers at Sutter have 25 percent
of their bonus pay based on achieving various quality initiatives.
Sentara's Resultshare program gives bonuses for performance
excellence (financial and customer satisfaction criteria) to all members of the organization. Bonuses range from 5 percent for all employees whose base pay is not at risk to 20 percent for managers
whose base pay is at risk. If the organization does not meet minimum criteria, no bonuses are paid out. Sentara executives also have
both short-term and long-term incentives in which 15 to 25 percent of their compensation pay is based on the system's meeting certain targets of which about one-third are quality targets.

Key to the success of these types of programs is a systematic
human resource planning process linked to the system's strategic
plan that identifies the needs and goals of the system (Williams,
1992). Training and development processes should foster integration by educating those involved to the desirability, concepts, and
methodologies of integration. Human resource practices that build
strong teams, reward team achievements on an ongoing basis, and
provide for management continuity promote overall integration.
Investment in cross-training employees and caregivers at all levels
should be expanded.

Sentara Healthcare views employees as a critical part of its business and has redesigned its human resource process to help produce
high-quality employees. First, the organization has developed a selection process that allows the system to identify potential employees with the appropriate service orientation. This includes a movie
regarding Sentara's values, a screening tool, and managers who are
trained to evaluate potential candidates. Sentara consolidated its
seven personnel centers into two and allows candidates to submit a
single application for all potential job sites. Sentara makes much

training available and subsidizes those who wish to continue formal education.

Sentara as well as a number of other systems are using 360 degree or 270 degree evaluation processes to some extent. Some departments at Sentara include information from customers, peers, subordinates, and/or superiors in the evaluation process. Franciscan Health System has found the 360 degree performance appraisal a very useful tool for improvement. An individual receives constructive feedback from those above and below, as well as at the same level, to help improve his or her performance. At this point the 360 degree technique is used for development purposes only, not for formal evaluation or payment, helping to take much of the fear out of this new process.

## Performance Assessment of the System

Integration is not easily assessed, but it is important to have a means of monitoring a system's progress in becoming integrated. In order to evaluate progress in the integration effort, systems can develop an "integration scorecard" that is shared throughout the system (Devers and others, 1994). Such a scorecard would track progress on specified measures over time. The measures would be linked to specific objectives and assigned to specific people and groups for purposes of accountability. Fairview has used a set of systemwide critical success factors, goals, and milestones that aid in assessment. Henry Ford has had several initiatives in this direction. It developed a comprehensive system performance profile that can be used to measure performance in four main areas: customer service, low-cost provider, system integration, and growth. (See Chapter Six for further discussion.) Baylor Health Care System has made the measurement of its performance part of its strategic plan; it specifies metrics by which progress toward various goals can be assessed. In the specification of its objectives, Mercy Health Services similarly specifies indicators and targets, as well as mean and methods by which the objectives can be achieved.

## Future Challenges and Issues

We argued in 1996 that the functional integration requirements of the organized delivery system (ODS) of the future are difficult to ascertain because the future health care world is uncertain. If anything, this uncertainty has increased, and the future is even less clear. It is not established where health care reform will lead; thus, ODSs must plan for a future that may hold unknown governmental requirements. Because the role of the ODS is to provide for the needs of the populations that it serves, it is likely that it will also need to change as the needs of the populations change. Finally, the changes the ODS will face in the future are likely to increase as technology changes the way medical care is delivered and those who deliver it.

The functional requirements of the health care system of the future are likely to be very different from those of today. A system will need to develop the functional support services necessary to manage populations over time. The functional infrastructure must also be able to meet increasing accountability demands, a burden that falls most heavily on the information systems and quality management functions of the organization. The functional infrastructure must be able to move from supporting inpatient acute care to primary care and care across the continuum, and it will have to adapt to communication technologies, biomedical science, and workforce changes. Finally, the functional infrastructure must simultaneously centralize and decentralize. For example, an ODS must be able to offer a common standard of care across its operating units but also allow for variations in treatments that are dictated by varying conditions. It must assign responsibility for the various functions to whichever levels—system, regional, or operating unit—add the greatest value to the system overall.

Successful health care systems in the future will be systems that promote learning and flexibility (Barnsley, Lemieux-Charles, and McKinney, 1998). They will be organizations that can make the complexity of the health care arena manageable and make the tasks seem not so overwhelming. Given the complexity and variety, no single model is likely to emerge. The process will continue to be one of trial and error. Nevertheless, some common themes will arise. Good communication among all the people touched by the system will be essential. Leaders will need to give consistent messages and follow through on their words. As one CEO said in an interview, people have to "realize that integration is not an option." Above all, system leaders must have patience because functional integration is a long, ongoing process. However, an organized delivery system must meet the challenges of functional integration in order to promote physician-system and clinical integration.

### Baylor Health Care System

In the early 1990s, Baylor Health Care System (BHCS) functioned as a multihospital system rather than an integrated health care delivery system. The organization included a tertiary teaching center, the Baylor University Medical Center (BUMC), which was designated as the system hub, and a ring of suburban community hospitals, specialty hospitals, and other related health care services that were designed to serve as "spokes" in support of the hub and the "wheel." Corporate support services and care delivery across the organization for the most part were not integrated.

Although the marketplace at that point did not require system redesign to improve care delivery and cost effectiveness, BHCS leaders decided that transforming Baylor into an integrated health care delivery system would better position the organization for managed care pressures that were anticipated in the late 1990s. The goal of the system redesign process was to offer well-coordinated delivery of high-quality, efficient, cost-effective services across the geography and across the BHCS continuum of care. The organization confronted a number of barriers to system redesign: its past success, a strong inpatient hospital focus, lack of a consistent organizational culture across all business units, and lack of a coherent and focused strategic vision.

In 1994 Baylor created the System Integration Action Team to develop and implement a plan for integrating clinical and nonclinical processes. This team was headed by the BHCS senior executive vice president/chief operating officer and consisted of twenty-eight Baylor clinical and nonclinical leaders. The team's initial efforts set out to define for the system the ideal core processes and to redesign a more efficient organization around those core processes. For fourteen months, the team planned, organized, and implemented system redesign concepts to improve organizational performance in an anticipated era of fixed payment. The team identified the ultimate end user or "customer" of the system as the patient. "Stakeholders," defined as those who have a great deal at stake in the ultimate success or failure of the organization, were identified as physicians, employees, volunteers, trustees, vendors, and other health care providers.

Team-defined core processes were designed first to meet the requirements of the customer and also to consider important requirements of system stakeholders:

- Manage illness—focusing on the patient and caring for the patient after injury or onset of illness

- Optimize health and wellness—keeping people healthy

- Coordinate patient education and access to care—managing initial and ongoing contacts with the patient or potential patient and facilitating access to system services

- Capture market—researching marketplace requirements, converting research findings into product and service designs, orchestrating the development of a network to deliver services, packaging products and services for contracting with health plans, and evaluating marketplace perceptions of system performance and value

- Assess and manage risk—managing all aspects of operational risk, including contracting risk, insurance risk, and organizational reputation

- Manage resources to support core processes—managing the infrastructure (information systems, human resources, financial services, material services, real estate and technology) required to support smooth functioning of the patient care processes in such a way that they are invisible to the customer

- Develop, update, and communicate BHCS objectives and strategies—identifying and prioritizing system initiatives and keeping the other six core processes informed of BHCS priorities for addressing requirements of the marketplace

System redesign efforts were focused on improving service quality outcomes, improving cycle time, reducing costs of service delivery, and increasing perceived overall system value. The redesign team committed to creating the capability for BHCS to make good decisions efficiently, communicate organizational direction to staff in a timely and meaningful way, and have organizational processes operating well enough to be first to market in addressing customer and stakeholder needs.

## Progress Toward Functional Integration

Having defined seven core processes, the Baylor team embarked on a multiyear project to reengineer the system into a fully integrated health care delivery machine. Design and implementation teams were created around each of the core processes, and many met the target date of January 1, 1997, for achievement of the system integration objectives. For example, BHCS efforts in the area of the seventh core process (develop, update, and communicate BHCS objectives and strategies) proceeded well. The team in charge of this core process created a distinctively new strategy development process that engages administrative and physician leaders in a collaborative effort to articulate and periodically update system priorities and to disseminate regular reports of progress to physicians and staff. Each system strategy is defined in measurable terms, contains multiyear targets, is led by a senior system leader, and is regularly tracked with reports of progress reported to an audience of thirteen thousand employees and fifteen hundred physicians across the system. In 1997, using the same survey instrument employed in the earlier Health Systems Integration Study, Baylor conducted its own assessment of the effectiveness of the thirteen elements of system integration and found that strategy development had improved remarkably at the system level.

The current BHCS strategic plan includes five high-level systemwide objectives and twenty-two supporting strategies. The objectives are measurable goals describing what BHCS must achieve within a given period of time in order to accomplish the organizational mission and vision for the future. The strategies define articulated courses of action through which BHCS hopes to achieve its objectives. Both the objectives and the relevant strategies have accompanying targets and metrics by which system progress is measured. As an example, the metric for Objective 1: Create and Enhance Alliances with Physicians is "physician commitment to BHCS," which is measured through a periodic survey of BHCS physician commitment to the organization.

Other areas of the system redesign effort have also made progress. In September 1999, BHCS hired the system's first chief scientist, an epidemiologist responsible for design and implementation of plans to improve population health through identification and implementation of processes to improve outcomes. In addition, clinical integration redesign work resulted in 1997 in the definition of eight systemwide clinical services lines (oncology, cardiovascular, neurology, pregnancy and childbirth, digestive disorders, respiratory, musculoskeletal, and diabetes) and the formation of interdisciplinary teams for each to design and deliver services focused on clinical quality, cost-effectiveness, and customer satisfaction. BHCS continues to work on the third core process, access to care, and has developed a promising model that is being field-tested in one community medical center before introduction to the system at large. The goal of this initiative is to facilitate consumer access to health care resources and simplify scheduling for services. Recent redesign of a systemwide "compliance" infrastructure and process has supported the organization's core process to "assess and manage risk." In terms of the sixth core process, "managing resources to support core processes," the financial services function has been redesigned to anticipate change more effectively and deliver financial services more efficiently. Information services is now guided by a new administrator-physician duo that has made good progress in creating an information services infrastructure and processes to support the other core processes. Human resources is one of the key processes yet to be redesigned.

## Obstacles to Integration

Although BHCS has enjoyed some success in achieving a more integrated approach to care delivery, system leaders are not as far along in redesign of the organization as they hoped they might be by now. Efforts to redesign the seven core processes have helped lessen the impact of some of the system integration barriers identified in earlier work of the Health Systems Integration Study. Some processes that were originally identified as deficient have been significantly improved. BHCS has also worked to develop a customer-focused, organizational culture that values physicians and staff members as the "Baylor family." During the past five years, BHCS's increased support of and attention to physicians and their perspectives has caused the system to develop a regional network of forty-one neighborhood, non-hospital-focused, outpatient health care centers that are conveniently located in "neighborhoods" that are close to consumer homes.

Although some of the obstacles to integration have been lessened and some successes have been achieved, BHCS leaders have found that the pace of anticipated progress has not tracked the original timetable. Several barriers, both old and new, have resulted in delays. For example, the organization continues to encounter staff members who do not understand or support system redesign efforts. And managed care pressures, although daunting, have not been successful in forcing health systems in the marketplace to rethink their approach to care delivery radically.

The major barrier to integration of BHCS, however, was its thirty-month merger discussions, now called off, with Texas Health Resources (THR), a merger of Presbyterian Health System and Harris Methodist Health Care System, to become the Southwest Health System. The proposed merger was viewed as an efficient means of providing easy access to a complete continuum of care for virtually all consumers in the metropolitan area. The initial merger talks that began in 1997 diverted the attention of BHCS senior leaders and brought system redesign efforts to a halt. The BHCS senior executive vice president and chief operating officer in charge of system redesign was reassigned as a key player in the merger discussions with THR. System energies and resources were redeployed from system redesign to address the proposed merger. When the merger talks broke off in the fall of 1999, BHCS had lost more than two years in its system integration effort.

## Keys to Success

Many of the factors that have helped Baylor become successful in the past will support its future system performance. Its forward-thinking leadership anticipates marketplace changes rather than responds to them. The organization's willingness to engage and involve physicians in positions of leadership and in decision-making processes has helped create relationships of trust between the system and physicians in the region, and those relationships, critically important to overall system performance, will continue to support system efforts to improve clinical care delivery, customer service, and cost-effectiveness. BHCS leaders have been persistent in their efforts to integrate their system. They have been willing to reexamine their plans and actions, change their approach as needed, and invest significant resources in efforts to improve system effectiveness.

## Lessons from the Baylor Experience

The BHCS system redesign experience highlights how each system's core processes are likely to vary depending on the organization's environment, mission, and values. The process of defining a system's core processes can help clarify its vision and its approach to achievement of that vision. It is a valuable learning experience that can be transferred to other areas. Defining core processes can also clarify what functions need to be integrated and which do not. An effort such as that of the Baylor System Integration Action Team, with its commitment of personnel and other resources, can help increase the visibility and heighten awareness of system integration goals.

Another lesson from the BHCS experience is that the energy required for an organization to consider and prepare for a merger is enormous. A potential merger siphons organizational resources and attention from other system priorities regardless of their importance. BHCS committed substantial leadership energy and focus to the merger effort and, as a result, drifted from some efforts to achieve a more integrated approach to delivery of health services.

## Future Directions

Once BHCS leaders decided to withdraw from merger discussions with THR, their attention was freed to focus on other priorities. The senior executive vice president, and now deputy chief executive officer, who headed the original system redesign effort has made system integration a renewed top priority for the organization. The ability of BHCS to differentiate its health care services from other providers in the marketplace is dependent on the success of the organization's ability to complete its original concepts for system redesign and integration.

◆　　◆　　◆　　◆　　◆　　◆

## Franciscan Health System

Franciscan Health System (FHS), headquartered in Tacoma, Washington, is an example of a proactive stance on health care that systems developed and implemented during this decade. At the beginning of the original Health Systems Integration Study in the early 1990s, FHS was known as Franciscan Health System West (FHS

West). It had operations in the Pacific Northwest, centering in the Washington South Puget Sound region and the eastern Oregon region. FHS West was the West Coast component of the Aston, Pennsylvania, corporation also known as Franciscan Health System, which included additional operations in Delaware, Maryland, New Jersey, and Pennsylvania.

## Progress Toward Functional Integration

In the early 1990s, FHS leadership made the conscious decision to focus system strategies on developing an integrated delivery network (IDN), defined as a patient care delivery system that offers care across the continuum. The entry of managed care into the market of the Northwest coupled with health care reform were two of the driving forces for this initiative. FHS's concentration of hospitals, developing physician network, and long-term facilities was the nucleus for delivering an integrative model of patient care.

The development efforts for an IDN at FHS focused on four key areas. The first area was developing management expertise: skill sets that allow organizations to compete effectively and efficiently in a given industry. Second, efforts focused on adding value—developing the network or service such that it is differentiated from others in the market by its innovative ways of delivering the goods or services that "add value" to the patient. The third area was developing capital access, obtaining the funds that are needed to support the strategic initiatives to achieve success. The final area was achieving sufficient leverage with suppliers and buyers to enable the organization to offer services in a cost-effective manner and improve earnings.

Under the leadership of its regional CEO, FHS aggressively pursued a course of "integration" through a one-board, one-management structure that permitted leadership direction across all acute care settings. Duplication of skills and roles was eliminated at all levels of management. The basic FHS management structure was centralized and organized by function, and a matrix style of management was implemented. Core competencies were developed and transferred within and across service lines in the organization, resulting in a number of best practices. Management and staff skills were multifaceted, and care teams became the model of service. The extent to which FHS was effective in eliminating duplication, achieving best practices through clinical effectiveness, eliminating waste, and improving quality all directly resulted in reduced cost to the patient, an achievement recognized by outside evaluators of health care performance. In 1994, St. Joseph Medical Center, the largest FHS facility, achieved recognition as one of the "nation's top 100 hospitals" from HCIA/ Health Network, an honor the hospital has continued to enjoy for six consecutive years. In 1999, St. Francis and St. Clare hospitals also received the top 100 hospitals award, making FHS the only health system nationally to receive this honor.

In 1996, Franciscan Health System joined two other Catholic health systems (Catholic Health Corporation of Omaha, Nebraska, and Sisters of Charity Health Care Systems of Cincinnati, Ohio) to become Catholic Health Initiatives (CHI). Because of its strong recognition in the Northwest with customers, and especially with payors, FHS retained its present name. This "new" FHS continued to pursue its consolidation strategy. A single medical staff was created. A CHI West entity was created and CHI delivery networks in Oregon, Washington, Idaho, and California were coordinated by this entity. This led to further economies of scale, transfer of best practices, and greater leverage with suppliers. About a year after CHI was formed, the CHI enterprise restructured, setting up four divisions headquartered in Denver, Colorado; Louisville, Kentucky; Aston, Pennsylvania; and Minneapolis, Minnesota, with FHS reporting to the Minneapolis office. The Denver office is CHI's corporate headquarters. It assists the component health systems by providing resource groups and solution teams in every functional area, serving as "national consultants" for the member health systems.

## Challenges to Integration

In the 1990s, FHS faced a number of challenges that had the potential to derail its integration efforts. First, the creation of CHI could have diverted focus from the integration strategy. FHS also experienced some turnover in leadership at both the top and middle levels. In addition, the introduction of matrix management required learning a new approach and set of skills. FHS also had to determine what would be the best distribution of functions for the system, that is, which functions should be primarily placed at the local, regional, and national levels. The mix of union and nonunion employees across independent employment sites within FHS made human resource issues even more challenging.

Similar to most of the other systems examined in this study, FHS had to develop relationships with its physicians that were acceptable to all involved. For example, the formation and ultimate dissolution of the employed primary care network, Medalia, put a huge financial and management strain on FHS. As in most other health systems, FHS had to focus much of its information system energies on Y2K issues. While it was successfully dealing with these Y2K challenges, however, many other aspects of its information technology strategy had to be placed on hold. In summary, all of these factors could have resulted in slowing or curtailing the development of the FHS integrated delivery network.

### Keys to Success at FHS

In spite of these potential challenges, FHS has been able to continue on its course toward integration. Many of the environmental factors identified in 1996 as encouraging the development of an IDN are still relevant for FHS. First, although revenue from managed care/risk contracting has stabilized at about 20 percent for the last several years, inherent efficiencies and low AAAPC rates in Washington state have jeopardized profit streams and encouraged continuous reduction of cost and variation across entities. The Balanced Budget Act of 1997 also applies pressure in this direction. And although physician integration has been slow, significant progress in cost reduction, clinical improvements, and referrals has been made with the primary care network, the hospital-based groups, and specialists.

A common challenge to many health care systems is determining which functions should be integrated and which should not be.

Through much thought and some trial and error, FHS has worked out a distribution of functions that works well for it. At this point, the vast majority of functions are performed at the local level. Geographic concentration of the FHS operating units (hospitals, physician groups, and long-term care centers) has assisted in integration. Other select functions such as cash management, insurance, legal services, purchasing, and consulting services are provided at the national level by CHI. This distribution of functions seems to be effective for FHS goals now, but system leaders are open to redistribution of functions should shifting trends in the environment or the system's strategy demand change.

Although not fully implemented yet, one factor facilitating FHS's integration efforts has been its use of 360 degree evaluation, in which those with direct-line as well as dotted-line responsibility give one another feedback. This evaluation process is supplemented with retreats at which the management and communication styles of the various members are discussed with an aim to extend constructive feedback. At this point, the 360 degree evaluation is not used to determine bonuses or performance. Rather, top system leaders are trying to implement the process as a learning tool, that is, to help teach individuals how to be better managers, improve communication, and work in a matrix organization. Thus far, it has been used only for the top management team, but it may eventually serve middle-line managers as well.

FHS's incentive compensation system also promotes system integration. Twenty percent of senior managers' salaries is at risk, based on achievement of two systemwide and two hospitalwide goals. A major portion (60 percent) of these bonuses is paid from the system's surplus. This means that if an individual hospital meets or exceeds its budget but the system does not, 60 percent of the bonus will not be awarded. This compensation system helps direct greater focus on the performance of the system rather than either the hospital or the individual.

Development of the clinical information system function is still in its infancy, but FHS is actively engaged in planning for its development. The development of its decision support system, on the other hand, began in the early 1990s. This system (called TSI) has been in operation for approximately five years and has become a system best practice, held up as a prototype for all of CHI. It provides high-quality, comparable data for effective decision making.

Franciscan Health System's commitment to values-driven, customer-focused TQM and the dissemination of this approach throughout the system has both augmented the traditional FHS culture and facilitated the integration effort. Efforts include FHS's "tools for teams," interdisciplinary teams, and a clinical effectiveness unit. These have been crucial for improvement in terms of both clinical and financial outcomes. For example, the clinical effectiveness unit tracks the amount of labor, services, equipment, medical supplies, and productivity to assess the efficiency of their efforts and make changes to increase that efficiency.

Strategic planning has become a significant strength of FHS; in a survey of some of the top system leaders at FHS, the rating of strategic planning was extremely positive. FHS has a three-year strategic plan that establishes four system goals, with tactics to accomplish the goals and specific measures to assess progress toward the goals. This plan was developed through a process that involved focus groups and hundreds of individuals, including managers, staff, physicians, and end users throughout the system. The resultant strategic plan is a guide to the goals of the system and helps maintain a consistent yet flexible focus on key leveraged activities.

## Lessons Learned

The FHS experience illustrates the importance of several factors, the first of which is culture. FHS's ability to respond proactively to the challenges that it has encountered is in part attributable to its strong values-based and TQM-based culture. The FHS experience also demonstrates the importance of strong leaders. Even if there is turnover in leadership, an organization can compete effectively and efficiently if those leaders who are present impart a consistent vision and possess strong skills.

Another key lesson from FHS is the need to establish a strategic plan that will ensure consistent focus for system efforts. Aligning incentives to support the strategic plan and system goals is also crucial. Finally, FHS has been successful because its board has supported difficult but necessary management decisions.

## Future Challenges

FHS continues to develop its integrated delivery network. Leaders are trying to strengthen matrix management throughout the system. They also are encouraging the assumption of greater intersystem responsibilities, especially by FHS's middle managers. But the major foci of the system are the goals defined in its 1999–2001 strategic plan. First, FHS wants to ensure that it is distinguished by its distinctive culture, based on compassion, service excellence, and innovation. Second, FHS strives to be a system of preeminent performance, especially in the areas of cardiology, general surgery, orthopedics, women's services, oncology, emergency, and endocrinology. FHS also is focusing on strengthening its physician relationships through trust and developing more innovative systems of care. The fourth goal involves enhancing advocacy and community health efforts. FHS leaders believe that their ability to plan as a system while staying flexible enough to respond to sudden changes in the environment will be the key to their future success.

# 4

. . . . . . . . . . . . . . . . . . . . . . . . . . . . . . .
,

# Physician Integration

P hysician integration is the extent to which physicians and the organized delivery systems with which they are associated agree on the aims and purposes of the system and work together to achieve mutually shared objectives. From a behavioral perspective, this is reflected in the extent to which physicians are economically linked to a system, use its facilities and services, and actively participate in its planning, management, and governance (Gillies and others, 1993).

The hospital-physician relationship has been an issue of long-standing investigation (cf. Pauly, 1980; Morrisey, Alexander, Burns, and Johnson, 1996, 1999; Shortell, 1991; Walston, Kimberly, and Burns, 1996; Burns and Thorpe, 1993). In 1996, 85 percent of all hospitals in the United States had formal relationships with physicians, an increase from 61 percent in 1993. More recently, attention has focused on physician-system relationships (Alexander and others, 1996a, 1996b; Zuckerman and others, 1998). This chapter presents some new evidence and observations on physician integration based on an update of the experiences of the study systems over the past four years, findings from a recently completed study of physician-system alignment issues, and a review of the current literature.

In our earlier work, we found modest levels of physician integration, with a mean value of 2.6 on a scale of 1 to 5 (from low to high) as perceived by numerous individuals (physicians and executives) associated with each system. Overall, however, the systems emphasizing more pluralistic approaches, such as the use of various combinations of owned physician groups, independent practice associations, physician hospital organizations, management service organizations, and the like, were further along in their physician integration efforts than systems focusing on a narrower range of initiatives. We also found that standardization of support services, such as human resources, information technology, strategic planning, and TQM, was positively associated with a greater degree of physician integration. Systems using "prospector" strategies emphasizing innovation and development of new services were further along in physician integration. A culture that emphasized teamwork and collaboration was also positively associated with physician system integration. Finally, we found that physician integration was positively associated with system total revenue and cash flow. This was particularly true with regard to the number of physicians who were practicing in groups. We also identified a number of external and internal obstacles to achieving physician integration and, based on our research at the time, highlighted some key success factors and examples of best practices. What has happened in the past four years?

## Recent Update

We collected data on each system's relationships with its physicians in regard to a variety of models: independent practice associations (IPA), closed physician hospital organizations (PHO), open PHO, management services organization (MSO), medical foundations, equity model, and the salaried model. We also asked about joint-venture activity, managed care contracting, physician credentialing, physician profiling, quality and outcome reporting, physician leadership and development training, and physician recruitment. In each case, we asked whether the model or activity was centralized at the systemwide or regional level, shared between these levels and an individual operating unit (such as an individual hospital), or decentralized at the operating unit level. We asked how satisfied the top management team was with their relationship or activity (1 = Not at all satisfied to 5 = Very satisfied), how important the activity was for achieving integration (1 = Not at all important to 3 = Very important), and the extent of implementation (1 = Just getting started to 3 = Fully implemented).

Most systems still use multiple models of physician-system integration, with the most prevalent being salaried group model, open-ended PHOs, and IPAs. No study systems were using equity models or closed PHOs, and only one was using the medical foundation model. Not surprisingly, the salaried group model tended to be centralized at system and regional levels, while the open PHO and IPA models tended to be more decentralized at the individual operating units. Satisfaction was higher for the salaried group and open PHO models than for the IPA and MSO arrangements. The salaried and open PHO models were seen as more important to the system's integration objectives than the IPA or MSO approaches. Respondents indicated that they were largely in the middle of their implementation efforts—beyond the just getting started stage but not yet at full implementation.

In regard to specific activities, physician leadership development and training and managed care contracting were most centralized, with all systems conducting these primarily at the systemwide or regional levels. Joint-venture activities and physician credentialing and profiling tended to be split, with some systems conducting these at the individual hospital level and others at the regional or systemwide level. Quality and outcome reporting also tended to vary from the individual hospital level to the regional and system level. The participating systems reported being moderately satisfied with all of the various activities (typically a 3 on the 1 to 5 scales) with the greatest degree of satisfaction expressed for managed care contracting. Managed care contracting and quality and outcomes reporting were each seen as most important to the system's integration objectives, followed by physician leadership development and training. Most of the activities were evaluated as moderately implemented, with quality and outcomes reporting receiving the highest implementation score.

As a whole, these findings indicate that most systems continue to take a pluralistic approach in their physician relationships, as found four years ago. The salaried group and PHO models are emerging as favored approaches. Most respondents were only moderately satisfied with their physician relationships and indicated that they were still in the middle stages of implementation. Some of the ongoing challenges to implementation arise from changes occurring within the medical profession at large, some from other factors in the external environment, and some from within the relationship of the hospital or health system to the physician.

## Continuing Evolution of the Medical Profession

To place these findings in context, it is important to understand the changes occurring within the medical profession at large. Organizations and professions are heavily influenced by their foundings and subsequent key events in their history. Values and norms defining appropriate behavior are often "imprinted" at birth and by key watershed events. In the case of medicine, the Hippocratic oath and the Flexner Report of 1910 have been the foundation stones of the profession. Many of the values expressed in the Hippocratic oath are timeless, have served well, and should be preserved across generations. Nevertheless, the social, economic, and political environment within which medicine is practiced has changed dramatically over the past three decades. Before that time, this environment was characterized by seemingly unlimited resources, high status and prestige for physicians and hospitals, a compliant and trusting population, generally favorable governmental legislation and regulation, and a generous payment system. But in the three past decades there have been increasing pressures to contain costs, focus more on population-based health care, be more responsive to consumers, and provide public accountability for quality and outcomes of care. The basis for trust is moving from a relatively uninformed public acceptance of professional expertise to one of evidence-based accountability. In the light of these dramatic changes, it is reasonable to ask whether the model within which the values of medicine are contained remains viable. Although the Flexner Report (1910) made an enormous contribution to upgrading and standardizing medical education based on the biomedical sciences, it was silent on the contribution of the social sciences and humanities. It may be time to reassess the status of medical education and health professions education at large. This is beyond the scope of this book, but it is important to recognize that the way in which physicians and other health professionals are trained is an important contextual factor influencing the ability of organized delivery systems to provide integrated patient care.

Perhaps the most fundamental change is the extent to which the profession has lost control over its work. Historians, sociologists, and other students of the professions have highlighted autonomy over one's work as a key defining attribute of a profession and have used the medical profession as the "ideal type" example (Abbott, 1988; Freidson, 1970a, 1970b; Scott, 1982; Starr, 1983; Stevens, 1971). For many reasons, the relative autonomy of the profession has been eroded and given way to countervailing forces at the federal, state, and community levels (Light, 1993; Hafferty and Light, 1995). Consequently there has been a demand for new and multiple forms of accountability on the part of physicians that in many respects they are ill prepared to perform (Shortell, Waters, Clarke, and Budetti, 1998). Unlike other sectors of American society, the medical profession largely skipped the industrial age and as a result is severely handicapped in attempting to adjust to its accountability and practice demands in the information age. The key achievement of the industrial age was the ability to achieve economies of scale and scope through mass production manufacturing techniques (Chandler, 1962). Medicine, however, remains largely a cottage industry. Even today, only 45 percent of physicians practice in groups, and 82 percent of these groups have fewer than ten physicians (Havlicek, 1999). It is extremely difficult, if not impossible, for those who are practicing in largely solo and small partnership practices to exchange information with colleagues; implement guidelines, protocols, and pathways; develop outcome measures demanded by purchasers; and keep up with the explosion of new medical knowledge.

Historically, most physicians relied on the voluntary hospital medical staff structure to meet some of their collective needs. But the hospital medical staff cannot meet the demands of managed care contracting and has given way to the new economic entities of PHOs, MSOs, and IPAs. This change has been exacerbated by the shift away from the hospital as the center of the delivery system as new technologies and payment systems created the means and the incentives for more care to be delivered on an outpatient basis, at home, or, increasingly, through the Internet (Shortell, Gillies, and Devers, 1995; Robinson, 1997).

The profound changes occurring within the medical profession are reflected in the comments of both young physicians entering the workforce today and by the collective voice of the American Medical Association (AMA). Most young physicians, for example, no longer talk about trying to "establish a practice." Instead, they try to "get a job" (Williams and others, 1999). At the collective level, the AMA recently passed a resolution supporting the unionization of physicians (Klein, 1999). Currently about forty-five thousand physicians (6 percent) belong to unions, a number that is expected to grow at a 15 percent annual rate over the next several years (Greenhouse, 1999, Havighurst, 1999; Scheffler, 1999).

We believe these changes reflect a profound restructuring of the medical profession to meet the challenges of the twenty-first century. At the center of this restructuring will be the profession's ability to redefine itself in relation to both patients and organizations. In regard to patients, this will require a sharing of power, democratization of the relationship, and accountability based on evidence. In regard to organizations, physicians can develop their own organizations, partner with an organized delivery system or network, or partner with physician practice management companies and health plans. Each has its advantages and disadvantages that will vary from market to market. What seems clear, however, is that current models and strategies based on managed care contracting are no longer adequate. What is needed are capabilities and relationships to manage care in a cost-effective fashion.

Effective medical practice will require an ability to be truly patient centered; ongoing capital investment; increasingly advanced information systems; the ability to work in teams; the ability to adapt to changes in treatment technologies, practices, and payment incentives; the ability to improve care continuously; and the ability to be responsive to external parties. The two fundamental factors to make all these happen are leadership and trust. Because these characteristics are so difficult to maintain on a consistent long-term basis, we believe the experimentation that we see today will continue well into this century (Begun and Luke, 1990; Robinson, 1999b). In the sections that follow we discuss what some leading organized delivery systems are doing to develop effective physician integration.

## External Barriers and Challenges to Physician Integration

The obstacles to achieving closer physician-system partnerships can be divided into those that are largely external to the organization and those that are primarily internal. The external are less susceptible to the direct influence or control of the organization than are the internal and will primarily require changes in public policy.

The two primary external factors influencing physician integration are the lack of common economic incentives and the presence of various legal and regulatory barriers.

### Lack of Common Economic Incentives

In most parts of the United States, hospitals and physicians do not experience the same financial incentives due to different forms of payment, including per diem, per case, fee for service, discounted fee for service, and capitation. Conflicting incentives are a particular problem for systems with pluralistic physician relationships ranging from salary to various fee-for-service models.

Capitation involves the payment of providers on per member per month basis to deliver a defined set of services to a defined group of enrollees. Of all the payment models, most believers believe it creates the greatest incentive for providers to work together toward common objectives. Full capitation of all components of the delivery system creates incentives for all parties—physicians, hospitals, and others—to manage resources prudently in regard to the production costs and the transaction costs of delivering care. Recent evidence suggests that provider capitation is one of the strongest factors promoting hospital-physician integration, particularly with regard to joint strategic planning, financial risk-sharing arrangements, and management services (Dynan, Bazzoli, and Burns, 1998). Yet capitation, particularly full capitation, has grown slowly and unevenly across the country, even in some highly penetrated managed care markets.

The lack of common economic incentives makes it extremely difficult for health system and physician leaders to build collaborative partnerships. In payment policy, as in most other things, Americans have choice and variety, but we may be underestimating the cost of those choices. The issue is whether the benefits outweigh the costs relative to what we are trying to achieve. It is important to note that the issue is *not* about a single-payer system; rather, in a *pluralistic*-payer system, would not more be gained by giving providers incentives for the up-front provision of care under a capitated budget and then holding providers accountable for both the fiscal and clinical outcomes of operating under that budget? For this to work on a widespread basis, two things must occur. First, continued advances must be made in the ability to adjust payments based on the health status of the enrolled population. Second, selected patient satisfaction, quality, and outcome measures must be incorporated into the contract to balance any tendency to withhold resources in which the benefits may outweigh the cost to patients. Until these occur broadly, misaligned economic incentives will continue to be a significant barrier.

### Legal and Regulatory Barriers

Efforts at physician integration can be hindered by state and federal laws and regulations. Some states, such as California, prohibit hospital ownership of medical groups. Also, tax-exempt financing guidelines may prohibit physicians from occupying more than 20 percent of corporate health system boards. In addition, federal antitrust legislation, if applied inflexibly, can prohibit mergers and consolidations of physician groups and physician groups with hospitals and other health care entities (Haas-Wilson and Gaynor, 1998; Kuttner, 1997; Hellinger, 1998; Liebenluft, 1999). The concern over anticompetitive pricing that may restrict consumer choice must be balanced against the opportunities for increased efficiencies and improved continuity and quality of care that might result from further consolidation of the system. For example, any willing-provider laws (allowing plans to contract with any physicians) would provide disincentives to IPA and group practice formation (Ohsfeldt, Morrisey, Nelson, and Johnson, 1998). Although these issues are not a major focus of this book, they are clearly important issues requiring careful assessment of the trade-offs involved.

## Internal Barriers and Challenges to Physician Integration

Most of the challenges to physician integration that we identified four years ago remain today. The exception is "satisfaction with the status quo." Most physicians throughout the United States now recognize that the practice of medicine will no longer be business as usual. The mantra of "fee-for-service leave me alone to practice medicine" is over. Dakota tribal wisdom says that when you discover you are riding a dead horse, the best strategy is to dismount. Some physician organizations are still trying to appoint a committee to study the dead horse or hire consultants to try to revive the horse or visit other sites to see how they ride dead horses; most physicians, however, realize the need to dismount, even if they do not know how.

The other barriers identified four years ago remain: fear and distrust, conflict between primary care physicians and specialists, lack of physician leadership, inadequate information systems, and lack of effectively functioning physician groups. Based on recent research, we identify a number of new subissues related to group practice, including lack of shared purpose, lack of shared culture, lack of strategic orientation, lack of meaningful physician input, and compensation issues.

### Fear and Distrust

Much of the fear and distrust that many physicians express is generalized distrust coming from the permanent structural changes occurring within the medical profession itself in response to societal forces. This is primarily related to the loss of clinical and practice autonomy and, as a result, a perceived lesser ability to control their professional careers. Most physicians' fear of large organizations is also a contributory factor.

Other aspects of physician fear and distrust are specifically related to existing relationships and experiences with local delivery systems. Goldsmith has colorfully captured these dynamics in the following statement: "Both sides of the bizarre, sadomasochistic relationship between physicians and hospitals bring baggage to the 'arranged marriage' of the integrated health system" (Goldsmith, 1993, p. 36). For example, at several of the study systems, physicians in small partnerships and group practices feared that the large, multispecialty group practices within the system would force themselves and their policies on the smaller groups and in effect take away their patients. In other cases, physicians feared that data on patient outcomes would be used against them. In another example, there was a general perception that the system was living "high on the hog" and not sharing the rewards of reduced hospital use with the doctors. In still another case, physicians felt they were viewed only as employees and not as integral partners. Also, distrust frequently existed among physicians themselves over who was promised what by the system and who was "getting more." These issues were exacerbated by the financial losses suffered by many physician groups—sometimes as much as $100,000 per physician per year.

It is also important to recognize that local community hospitals are no longer able to serve the role of being the physician's organizational security blanket since the key decisions are now being worked out between economic units of physicians and larger health systemwide entities such as PHOs, MSOs, and IPAs. These new arrangements are based on economic, legal, and managerial parameters that are still unfamiliar to many physicians and thus promote anxiety. The difficulty of integrating physicians is particularly pronounced in systems in which some key hospitals still enjoy significant autonomy and use it to try to reinforce physician linkages with the hospital rather than with the system (Shortell and others, 1993). This greatly restricts the ability to develop sharing arrangements across practices and operating units and to spread best practices across the system.

Insight into the relationship between physicians and health systems can be gleaned by considering the physicians' trust in the system on the one hand with the physicians' degree of control on the other hand, as shown in Figure 4.1. Cell 1, which represents the healthiest relationship between the physicians and the system, is characterized by physicians' perceiving that they have a high degree of control and a high trust relationship in the system. Cell 2 shows a relationship between physicians who perceive that they have little control but also perceive a high degree of trust in the system. These are characterized as "vendor" relationships and are found in the case of some salaried primary care groups. As long as the group continues to trust the system, this can be a viable relationship. In cell 3, physicians perceive they have a great deal of control but little trust in the system. In this situation, they can make attempts to dictate to the system and

Figure 4.1. Physician-System Relationships.

|  | | Physician Perceived Degree of Control | |
|  | | HIGH | LOW |
| --- | --- | --- | --- |
| | HIGH | Healthy, Productive Relationship | Vendor Relationship |
| Physician Level of Trust in the System | LOW | Dictating Relationship | Resentful Bondage Relationship |

impose their demands. Cell 4, the most dangerous situation, is characterized by low control and low trust in the system; physicians in this situation find themselves in a position of "resentful bondage."

Most of the study systems had relationships with physician organizations in all four of the cells depicted. Physicians in the "resentful bondage" cell were generally pushing for more control and autonomy so that they could dictate to a system that they did not trust, while the health systems, for their part, were trying to push the physicians into a vendor relationship that the system could control. Based on impressions gained from site visits, we believe that systems and physicians that were working toward both more physician autonomy over their own practices and more trust in the system to be good partners were making more progress in developing sustainable relationships.

## Conflict Between Primary Care Physicians and Specialists

There are naturally occurring differences between primary care physicians and specialists (as well as within these two groups) as a function of career interests, educational experiences, preferences for different kinds of patients, income, and other related factors. The current economic environment intensifies these differences as primary care physicians and specialists see themselves competing for patients while trying to change practice styles in the process. More important, the relative power of specialists has diminished as primary care physicians have assumed a more central role as the initial contact point with patients and as major decision makers regarding referrals to specialists and sites of care throughout the system (Grumbach and others, 1999). This relative power shift is accentuated by a shortage of primary care physicians in some cases and a rather marked oversupply of specialists in nearly all cases. In response, some specialists have organized their own specialty niche services in such areas as cardiology, oncology, and orthopedics (Berg, 1999).

Given this situation, systems face a tough challenge in attempting to bring primary care physicians and specialists together to accept risk. The issues involve how the capitated dollar is divided, criteria for patient referral, the appropriate use of primary care physicians and specialists in managing chronic illness, and the adoption and implementation of agreed-on clinical guidelines and outcome measures. New relationships with specialists must be formed that appropriately recognize their contribution to the economic viability of multispecialty groups.

## Lack of Physician Leadership

Initiating and implementing the changes to deal with the turbulent forces in health care environment require concerted leadership by all parties. In this regard, physician leadership has frequently been a missing link in the health care chain (Hughes, 1994). Most physicians understandably are interested in practicing medicine and generally have a distaste for administrative or managerial concerns and the time required to address these concerns. However, as professional work is increasingly practiced in complex organizations enmeshed in turbulent environments, there is a need for professionals to assume broader leadership and managerial roles. The first generation of physician leaders generally received little management training and focused their attention primarily on individual institutions, departments, or divisions. Typical examples were the hospital vice president for medical affairs, the director of medical education, or the chief of a specific service line or division.

A second generation of physician leadership is beginning to emerge that focuses on a broader range of health care delivery. These physicians, who are beginning to receive more systematic training, are assuming systemwide responsibility for clinical integration, quality improvement, and group practice management (Dunham, Kindig, and Schulz, 1994). Their training ranges from two- to four-day intensive courses to summer courses to, in some cases, M.B.A.s and related master's degrees in health services management. These individuals must overcome significant obstacles to become effective executives, not the least of which is their marginality in terms of being neither fully accepted by their colleagues—who will view them as having sold out to administration—nor fully accepted by their nonclinical managerial colleagues, who may view them as threats, intruders, or Johnny-come-latelies.

There is a need for a third generation of leadership in which all physicians in medical school and residency programs learn some basic managerial and leadership skills in communication, conflict management, change management, team building, and continuous improvement methodologies in order to be better prepared to practice in a changed environment and accept as well as contribute to new leadership approaches. A subgroup of these physicians will need to choose clinical careers that combine medicine and management in helping to restructure the delivery system. The current Flexnerian-based approach to medical education needs to include more content in the social, behavioral, and managerial sciences.

By the same token, nonclinical managers and executives need broader exposure to clinical management issues and population-based health care delivery models and greater understanding of the developing advances in the biomedical sciences. More managerially informed clinicians and more clinically informed managers are needed to make the changes required.

From a recent study of physician group practices affiliated with organized delivery systems, it is evident that significant leadership challenges remain (Shortell, Zuckerman, and Gillies, 2000). In most groups, the leadership is at best skin deep, composed of a few individuals. Not only does this hinder relationships between the group and the system, but it also impedes the ability of different clinics or practice sites within the group to transfer best practices. The overall situation is best reflected by field notes based on a visit to one system: "Physician leadership has not been fostered by [the system]. Physicians feel their voice isn't heard by [the system's] management. There are no physicians at high levels in [system] management."

### Inadequate Information Systems

A major operational barrier to physician integration is the lack of information systems that connect patients, providers, and health plans across the different settings of care. These systems are needed not only to provide access, cost, quality, and outcome data for external accountability purposes but also to meet CQI objectives and to provide the ability to track patients and populations over time. The exchange of information is at the center of the physician-patient relationship, yet relative to other fields, health care spends little on this fundamental process, constituting slightly less than 2 percent of operating budgets versus 6 to 7 percent in other fields (Dorenfest and others, 1995). But money alone is not the answer. Caregivers and managers need to do a better job of delineating what the information is for, what type of information is useful, and how the information can best be turned into knowledge and, indeed, wisdom in serving patient and community needs. Also, greater attention needs to be given to data confidentiality issues and the development of national standards for clinical information. The implications of the expanded consumer use of the Internet for medical information also need to be recognized.

Field notes from the study of the fifty-five physician groups underscore the above needs:

There seems to be a lack of coordination between systemwide and physician-level efforts. Many of the information systems, especially the clinical information systems, are old and cumbersome.

Although the system has allocated substantial resources to information technology development, the information systems do not yet reflect this spending. Some physicians complained that even voice mail was only now slowly being connected.

The information systems staffs from each entity do not appear to be working together or communicating frequently about issues of common interest. Information systems strategic planning does not appear to be a joint effort on the part of the medical group and the system.

Lack of information systems is a barrier to physician alignment. The system expanded rapidly four years ago and acquired physician groups without having the infrastructure to truly align them. As a result, there is not common billing, tracking of outcome measures, patient satisfaction, or quality assurance.

### Group Practice Formation Issues

We view the formation of effective group practices as probably the largest single barrier to physician integration. It is difficult to imagine a significant degree of physician integration occurring without more physicians' practicing in some form of grouplike arrangement. There are many potential advantages to physicians, systems, and patients alike:

- Expanded coverage of given geographic markets in order to capture greater numbers of patients

- Better coordination of patient care and provision of more cost-effective care through the use of guidelines, protocols, pathways and related care management practices

- Achievement of some economies of scale with the ability to spread overhead costs

- Improved communication between physicians and other members of the health care team

- Better teamwork and coordinated patient care as a result of transferring learning and best practices more quickly

- A sufficiently large patient base on which to collect reliable and valid functional health status, patient outcome, and patient satisfaction data

Groups can also increase physicians' sense of control over their professional careers and provide some degree of psychological security.

But the potential is at least matched by the challenges of implementation. Among the most important are these:

- Lack of a shared purpose, aim, or vision

- Lack of a shared culture

- Lack of a strategic orientation

- Lack of meaningful input into decision making

- Problems associated with different compensation and payment models

*Lack of a Shared Purpose: "Is That What We're All About?"*

Many physician integration arrangements were put together for economic and financial reasons related to managed care contracting and expansion of patient volume. This has been true for health systems and physicians alike. Relatively little emphasis has been given to how these arrangements might benefit patients and create longer-run value. The transactions have essentially been defensive, preemptive "knee-jerk" responses to payer pressures and consolidation of health plans. In many cases, the arrangements were designed to preserve the status quo. Some comments from the recent fieldwork notes are illustrative:

> Governance of the group is more of a defensive posture, with members protecting what they have.

> The infrastructure was designed to maintain the status quo, not built for change.

> Clinics have tended to operate as independent entities, not as part of a coordinated network.

> Typical of many physician groups, only a relative small proportion of the group membership participates in committee meetings.

> There is no common policy of referrals for the primary care physicians. Some can refer out of the system, and others cannot.

> Many of the physician groups appear to be very loosely organized. The practice sites rather than groups per se represented their primary orientation. In some cases, central billing and collection is the only shared activity within the group.

*Lack of a Shared Culture: "Walls Without Group Practices"*

For the most part, medical groups are groups in name only. They share few of the attributes associated with a group such as a sense of shared belonging, shared psychological identity, common values and expected behavior as reflected in certain clinical practices and policies, and shared information systems and reporting practices. Most lack a basic sense of collaboration. To our surprise, these were issues for long-established groups as well as those more recently formed, as the following field notes at one long-established but growing group practice noted:

> The group is more concerned with its survival than the need to integrate. The relatively rapid growth over recent years has led to a heterogeneous physician culture with multiple and sometimes conflicting values and beliefs. In spite of efforts to reduce or eliminate tensions, divisions continue to persist among differing sets of physicians.

Most health systems and physician leaders alike underestimate what it takes to develop a culture that fosters some common values that can be implemented in daily practice. Anyone and everyone can give lip-service to quality and excellence in patient care, but we are talking about coming to agreement on how professionals are going to work together to implement high-quality, cost-effective patient care. Physicians are highly individualistic even when practicing in small groups of four or five. To attempt to bring these groups into a larger practice entity is a significant challenge (Bollinger, 1999).

Most groups in the United States today have been cobbled together from smaller groups or partnerships or even solo practices. Said one system CEO about a group: "This was never really a group. It was really more a collection of small practices. They had really never done any consolidation of sites or created a group culture among those physicians. So it was a group in name only and there were a lot of inefficiencies built into the way they were operating."

The stark fact is that for the most part, these physicians are entrepreneurially oriented men and women who want to practice medicine. They increasingly recognize the economic necessity of being a part of some larger unit but see this primarily as a necessary evil as opposed to being a desired feature of their professional career. Upon completing seventeen site visits over the past two years to medical groups across the country ranging in size from six to over one thousand and covering all practice types, we reached this conclusion: "When you think you have seen one medical group, you *haven't* seen one medical *group*."

A few years ago, Sutter Health System, based in Sacramento, California, coined the phrase "group practice without walls" (GPWW) to reflect loosely organized, decentralized groups of physicians who practice at various medical campuses throughout the community. Based on our interviews of over four hundred physicians and executives in the seventeen group practice sites over the past two years, we believe we have discovered a new dominant practice model in the United States. We call it *walls without group practices* (WWGPs). It may well serve as the gold standard for virtual integration. The following summaries from our field notes are illustrative.

The system may choose to acquire a physician practice to forestall acquisition of that practice by a rival group or system. The system would then require these doctors to be incorporated into the larger group without regard to clinical or cultural fit.

There does not seem to be one culture but rather an amalgam of the individual cultures of the various groups making up the system. Physician leaders tend to be focused on getting what is best for the individual clinics (or even the individual physicians) rather than pursuing mutual system goals.

This physician organization doesn't yet have a unified culture and an agreed-on set of common values. Its culture was described by some as a "loose tribal affiliation"

Given the group's size and the way it has grown (largely through acquired practices), the group does not yet have a coherent sense of self or a shared culture.

Some of the lessons about the importance of cultural fit have been learned by the study systems. The CEO of one group commented:

We are still adding physicians to our foundation model and will continue to do so. But we are much more careful now than we were before. We first look at the physician culture of the group we are thinking of taking on. We ask whether their objectives are the same as what we are trying to accomplish with our other groups. You can't build the economic model first and then try to fit the culture. That's why for every ten physician groups that come to us, we only take on two.

*Lack of a Strategic Orientation: "What's a Strategy?"*

Many efforts to build physician integration are done for short-run defensive reasons of capturing physician practices before competitors do. Relatively little consideration is given to the compatibility of the group with the system's long-run strategic objectives. Nor are most physician group practices themselves strategic in their thinking or orientation. They tend to focus on short-run financial viability, and even here, management is often by instinct and lacks fundamental financial controls. Again, field note summaries provide relevant examples.

System input is mostly global. They generally take a "one size fits all" approach.

There is inadequate consideration of how network development will impact the group.

Clinics have tended to operate as independent entities, not as part of a coordinated network.

Physician acquisition/affiliation of practices are not well tied to the overall strategic plan of the system. Neither is there a primary care strategic plan for the system that is clearly communicated to the group.

We went out and bought anything that breathed, and that was a mistake. The doctors don't know each other, and that's a barrier to greater integration of the groups and alignment with the physicians.

Many of the physicians do not seem to be oriented to the business aspects of their practices. Few indicated that they do much strategic planning, although at least one group has contracted with a consulting firm.

*Lack of Meaningful Physician Input: "Where Is My Voice?"*

Many of the earlier models of physician integration were characterized by ritualistic physician involvement but little real input. In the past few years, there has been considerable movement toward more shared decision making between health systems and physician organizations. This is reflected in the governing boards of physician organizations dominated by physicians and the increased numbers of physicians on the governance of the health system board, plus the increased numbers of physicians in influential management positions throughout the system. As one CEO stated, "The physicians need to be involved in the shared decision-making process. If you have missed that, you have missed it all." Nonetheless, the lack of such involvement in many cases remains a barrier. Some illustrative examples from our fieldwork are highlighted:

Physicians feel their voice isn't heard by system management. There are no physicians at high levels of management.

Management thinks like hospital administrators. They try to tell physicians to do X, Y, and Z because we say so. They don't see the physicians as integral partners. They see them as employees.

*Compensation Issues: "I Don't Really Understand How I Am Paid"*

The lack of an external reimbursement environment that promotes aligned incentives contributes to chaos in the design and implementation of payment mechanisms for physician groups and systems in local markets. Although there has been a movement away from both straight or pure salary on the one hand and fee-for-service on the other, no one knows exactly how best to meet in the middle. A great deal of experimentation is occurring and will continue to occur, particularly in regard to incentives to encourage both productivity and prudent use of resources on the one hand and incentives for patient satisfaction, quality, and outcomes of care on the other. A few systems are experimenting with gain-sharing programs, whereby any savings generated from more cost-effective practices are shared with the physicians. Although the legality of these programs is being debated, these programs are likely to be short lived unless they can be tied to long-run, ongoing strategic objectives of the system related to value creation. Also, they need to be part of a system's overall gain reward system that involves executives and employees in addition to physicians. A program for physicians alone will be resented by others. More important than any particular model that is advanced is the process used. The process must be seen by physicians as fair and open, with considerable involvement at all stages. Some illustrative comments regarding the compensation issues are reflected in the following field notes:

The increased focus on productivity and budgets is eroding some of the mutual trust. This is seen by physicians as a statement that they are inefficient and not working hard.

One of the problems is that it is hard to count capitated revenue lives in the compensation scheme. The actions of physicians lower length of stay significantly, but they don't see the gains from that; the hospital does.

The current incentives are trivial. One cannot incent a business unit that is losing money.

While the primary care specialist physician compensation formula has apparently been successfully resolved, agreement on the secondary care specialist physician formula has yet to be accomplished. There is great potential for discord not only with the secondary care physicians if they do not get what they deserve but also if the primary care physicians think the secondary care physicians get more than they deserve.

Some of the agreements between physicians and the previous administration were individual verbal agreements. Current administrators still come up against these side agreements, such as "a former vice president promised me $x$ not to leave."

Production standards are based on medical group management association (MGMA) national benchmarks. Local physicians do not accept application of these national standards to their situation.

Physician compensation mechanisms have been a barrier because they vary widely among physicians, and they are not aligned properly with incentives. In the mad rush to acquire physicians in the beginning, the employed physicians receive large base salaries based on projected earnings, and most physicians increased their salaries.

## Key Success Factors

The key success factors for promoting physician integration have crystallized over the past four years. As shown in Figure 4.2, they are related to the ability to manage patient care risk. We distinguish between patient care risk and insurance risk. Physicians and health systems should not be held responsible for insurance risks reflected by differences in the age, sex, and initial health status characteristics of the enrollees. To the extent possible, these should be taken into account in the population-based risk-adjusted payment formulas. After these adjustments are made, physicians and health systems should expect to be held accountable for the cost, quality, and outcomes of care for their enrolled populations. This would be true regardless of whether capitation grows as a dominant form of payment because purchasers—private and public alike—will continue to push to contain cost while trying to maintain choice and access to new diagnostic and treatment advances. As a result, the key capabilities or success factors are those related to the ability to manage patient care risk.

Using our updated interview information and analysis of documents, along with the recently completed study of fifty-five physician groups associated with fifteen organized delivery systems (six of these organized delivery systems were in our earlier study) and our review of relevant literature, we have identified five characteristics that directly affect the ability to manage patient care risk:

- Aligning financial incentives

- Implementing new care management practices

- Promoting the evolution of effective information technology

- Accelerating and expanding CQI capabilities

- Moving toward population-based health care delivery models

Figure 4.2.  Key Success Factors for Physician Integration.

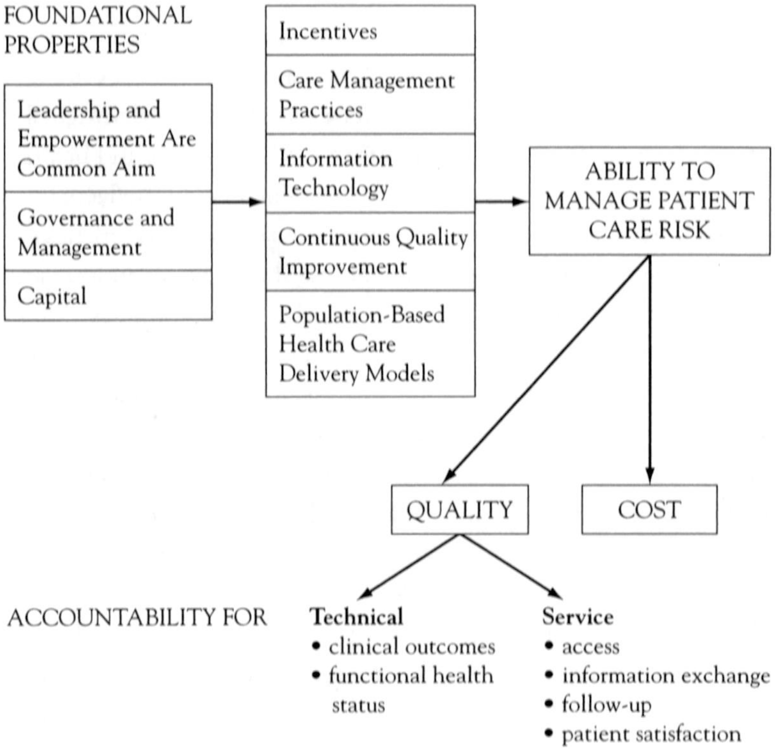

FOUNDATIONAL PROPERTIES

| Leadership and Empowerment Are Common Aim |
| Governance and Management |
| Capital |

| Incentives |
| Care Management Practices |
| Information Technology |
| Continuous Quality Improvement |
| Population-Based Health Care Delivery Models |

ABILITY TO MANAGE PATIENT CARE RISK

QUALITY          COST

ACCOUNTABILITY FOR

**Technical**
• clinical outcomes
• functional health status

**Service**
• access
• information exchange
• follow-up
• patient satisfaction

We also identified three characteristics that serve as a foundation for developing these five capabilities:

• The leadership and empowerment needed to develop a common aim or purpose

• Governance and management capabilities

• Capital

Absent from these characteristics is any discussion of specific models of physician-system integration—whether they are looser forms such as IPAs, intermediate forms such as PHOs or MSOs, or tighter forms such as equity models, foundations, and salaried staff models. Our experiences and those of others (Alexander and others, 1996a, 1996b; Bodenheimer, 1999; Robinson, 1999b) suggest that each of these forms has advantages and disadvantages depending on local market circumstances and the historical evolution of relationships in local markets. We believe that a more fruitful approach is to dig deeper and try to identify certain core features of these relationships that may be common across models. We view these as robust properties in the sense that they are likely to be approximately correct or promotive of effective integration regardless of specific models used or changes in the external environment (Shortell, Waters, Clarke, and Budetti, 1998).

### Robust Properties of Physician Integration

Each of the five capabilities we identify as robust properties for managing patient care risk are discussed in turn below.

#### Aligned Incentives

"Only those physicians at financial risk will change their practice patterns, and they will need to see the need for change before they will embrace change. And for that, of course, you need to align the incentives"(Eddy, 1999). To this cogent observation, we would add that physicians need to be convinced that it is the right thing to do for their patients based on evidence and experience and, often, with a healthy dose of peer pressure. But aligned financial incentives are a necessary condition for change to occur.

Regardless of how the health plan or overall physician organization is paid, individual physicians must be compensated in a way that facilitates making risk trade-off decisions: between prevention and treatment and between a single individual and the enrolled population at large. We know of no magic formula to accomplish this. But there are some important principles that should be followed.

First, the compensation incentives, however constituted, should be spread across a reasonable number of physicians so as to reduce the tendency for the individual physician to use fewer services because the direct financial gain is so apparent and immediate. An opposite problem, of course, is created when incentives are placed on such a large number of physicians that no one feels he or she can benefit from individual actions to use resources more prudently. As a rule of thumb, based on our experience in working with the study systems, providing direct incentives for a group of physicians as small as five or six doctors is probably too small, and placing them at the level of two hundred or more physicians is probably too large. Empirically documenting a useful range is a major area for further research.

Second, the compensation incentives should include a combination of productivity, patient satisfaction, technical and service quality, and leadership and good citizenship behaviors. Although many groups have learned the problems of paying on a 100 percent salary basis, the opposite extreme of paying on 100 percent productivity creates problems of churning and can lead to lower patient satisfaction and physician burnout. Depending on the strategic objective of the partnership, most systems are experimenting with a combination of productivity, quality, resource use, and citizenship factors. "Blended" payments based on a combination of capitation and fee-for-service are also being considered (Robinson, 1999a). The field notes provide a flavor for this experimentation:

> Emphasis on productivity-based compensation has advantages. Some sites compare their productivity with MGMA for benchmarking purposes. They are also beginning to build in quality criteria.

> A limited set of pilot incentive programs have tried to tie incentives to performance at department levels. All of them failed to pay out. One of the things that we have learned is that participants in these incentive schemes have to have the ability to control the outcomes. Otherwise, they fail.

The compensation system, while in place for less than a year, appears to be successful in reducing physician grievances about inequality and raising production as measured by relative value units and gross revenue generated. Revenues were raised by 30 percent over the past year. The strengths of the compensation systems were seen as its simplicity and its emphasis on paying for production.

Compensation is almost entirely productivity based rather than salary based. But patient satisfaction data are collected, and clinic level feedback is provided quarterly.

Although there remain issues to be addressed, the compensation system does attempt to strike a balance in its components by including not only productivity but also other attributes, such as teaching, research, and having a team orientation, which are valued by the system. Further, the compensation system is physician driven and administered.

A third principle, basic to compensation arrangements in any sector, is that incentives should be applied only to those areas in which physicians can control the outcome. Physicians should not be held responsible for things that are largely out of their control. As more health care is delivered in teams, this will become an increasingly difficult criterion to meet. For example, how much of patient satisfaction scores can be attributed to the physicians' office staff? How much of a functional health status score can be attributed to the overall team caring for the patient as opposed to a specific individual physician? The performance criteria must be very carefully targeted to each physician's domain of practice. This, of course, will vary by specialty, and often within specialty, and represents a major challenge to physicians' perceptions of equity.

A fourth principle is that the entire process must be seen as fair, just, and open. Research in other fields suggests that people will accept some degree of unequal payment and rewards if they believe that the decision-making process was open and fair and had their involvement (Lind and Tyler, 1988). It is also important that these arrangements be seen as an ongoing experiment with the opportunity to revise as experience is gained.

Our experiences and those of others suggest a number of characteristics that most physicians desire in constructing a financial relationship with their health system partners (Shalowitz, 1994; Shortell and others, 1996):

- Establish a sufficient volume of patients to diffuse risk, or use creative payment schedules until the risk threshold targets are met.

- Provide timely and accurate eligibility data, preferably through on-line computer linkages.

- Set capitation based on realistic risks and allow compensation for adverse selection.

- Provide appropriate stop-loss insurance and first-dollar reinsurance—the latter for high-risk cases such as open heart surgery and selected psychiatry and chemical dependency conditions.

- Help obtain favorable supplier contracts.

- Leave the physician alone to manage his or her own practice—that is, do not micromanage care.

- Provide assistance in implementing guidelines, conducting clinical outcome studies to improve care, and developing outcome data for purposes of external reporting.

- Share profits as befits a true partnership and a true risk-reward relationship.

These points are well summarized in the comments of one system: "Sharing the benefits of partnership will only happen if a system is integrated financially and economically. The more economically aligned incentives are, the better it will be."

*Care Management Practices*

At the core of the ability to manage patient risk is the ability to make changes in the way in which medical and health services are delivered. Care management practices refer to the use of evidence-based guidelines, protocols, pathways, case and care management systems, disease management systems, demand management, and related approaches. The goal is to reduce unnecessary variation in clinical practices and thereby improve quality and outcomes of care for the same or lower cost. Although much has been written about the need to change clinical practice, our findings suggest that these efforts are relatively embryonic. For example, in a recent study of fifty-five medical groups associated with most of the current study systems, the average number of conditions for which one or more care management practices were being used was approximately two (Budetti and others, 2000). Further, most sites could not report the percentage of eligible patients actually being cared for with the particular care management practice. The most frequent activity was reported for asthma, diabetes, congestive heart failure, and depression. But even here most of the focus was on the acute inpatient phase of the treatment continuum for these conditions rather than being applied across the continuum of care.

There are, of course, many barriers to changing clinical practice, not the least of which is the problem of getting physicians to adopt a specific guideline or protocol when only a small percentage of their patients are associated with the health plan or the system promoting the protocol. Most physicians, even those primarily affiliated with a single system, had patients who belong to different health plans or systems. These physicians understandably asked the following question: "Why should I use your protocol or guideline when I get only 15 percent of my business from you and others are also asking me to use their protocol and guidelines?" We found as a general rule of thumb that approximately 30 percent of a physician's practice needed to come from a single source before the physician would consider adopting that source's recommended care management practices. Thresholds appear to be as important as "withholds" in modern medical management.

Some systems are making more progress than others in implementing new care management practices. They tended to be those that had strong physician leadership, long-standing experience with and commitment to CQI, somewhat more advanced clinical information systems, and either owned or had a strong affiliation with a health plan that provided a nucleus of patients to the physicians. Some examples are reflected in the following summary field notes:

> The system's extensive use of case managers to work with high-risk patients is a better practice. They use primary teams composed of one primary care physician, a case manager, and a pharmacist. Some of their primary care physicians are open to alternative or complementary therapies and are actively integrating them into traditional care.

> The system has a number of exemplary clinical care management models, particularly in areas of behavioral health, occupational medicine, and formulary management.

> The creation of a care management institute facilitates the coherent development of care management practices. It has implemented selected community-based care management for certain chronic conditions.

> The role of the care integrator seems to be very beneficial for the development and implementation of care management practices.

The "inpatient manager" set up a hospitalist function well. Having separate physicians managing the inpatient care makes the ambulatory care more efficient.

There is obvious support for the development and implementation of care management practices. For example, selected physicians during the past year have been given two days off a week in order to work on implementing new care management practices.

Some of the physician groups have involved representatives from all levels in the development of their care management practices, thus gaining buy-in through the development process.

### Information Technology

In our earlier work, information technology was identified as among the least integrated functions of the study systems. It remains a major barrier at the same time that its importance over the past four years has grown given the demand for greater external reporting and accountability. Most study systems have learned the lesson, however, that an investment in information technology is not likely to pay off unless one first has in place a common aim and purpose for the physician integration relationship (that is, a shared strategic purpose), committed leadership, and an understanding of the information needs and requirements of all major providers within the system. If these are not in place, the implementation of information technology flounders. Even when these are in place, the capital requirements for information technology investment are daunting, and the time needed for return on these investments is generally longer than for other types of investment. More than one study system has had to pull back or delay capital investments in information technology due to unanticipated operating losses (in part resulting from the impact of the Balanced Budget Amendment of 1997) and preparations required for dealing with the Y2K challenge.

Most systems are currently using an incremental strategy based on implementing computerized patient records in selected physician offices. Typically this begins with a couple of offices, and as experienced is gained, additional practice sites are brought along.

*Accelerating Continuous Quality Improvement Capabilities*

CQI goes hand in hand with information technology and care management practices as a requirement for the ability to manage patient risk. The ability to improve care and add value continuously depends on a thorough understanding of current care management practices and then being able to collect and analyze the data and information to change those practices as needed. These changes are not only at the level of a specific clinical guideline or protocol but also at the level of reconfiguring the overall size and structure of the physician organization itself and its relationship to the system. For example, Kaiser/GroupHealth Cooperative of Puget Sound sees more of its diabetes and asthma patients in groups than in individual office visits. Kaiser Permanente's headquarters office in Oakland, California, has developed a care management institute to identify and diffuse evidence-based new practice methodologies more rapidly throughout the Kaiser Permanente system and anticipate how medical care will be practiced ten years from today. Nearly all of the study systems have developed the equivalent of an institute or center for clinical effectiveness to serve as an applied research and development laboratory and technical assistance center for the quality improvement work of providers. As clinical work is restructured, study systems and their associated physician groups are realizing that CQI also has significant implications for staffing and health manpower policy. This is reflected in an increased use of hospitalists (Wachter and Goldman, 1996; Wachter, 1999) to manage inpatient care and in the case of care managers (typically nurses) to manage patients across the continuum of care.

Although there is relatively little systematic evidence to show a payoff from investments in clinical quality improvements to date, some of the conditions for its success are beginning to be identified (Blumenthal and Kilo, 1998; Shortell, Bennett, and Byck, 1998; Institute of Medicine, 2000a). Also, there is some evidence that progress is being made in the clinical application of CQI in hospitals across the country. For example, recent data show that 93 percent of reporting hospitals are active users of CQI in some form, with significant increases between 1993 and 1998 in the percentage of physicians, managers, and staff trained in CQI processes; there is also increased participation in quality improvement teams and a greater number of perceived statistically significant improvements in patient outcomes (Arthur Andersen and the American Hospital Association, 1999a).

*Population-Based Health Care Delivery*

Managing risk means helping to manage the health of enrolled populations. Everyone benefits by keeping people well. When illness or injury strikes, everyone benefits by the prudent use of necessary resources to restore the patient's health. Practicing population medicine requires learning to make trade-offs wisely.

Two trade-offs are particularly important. The first is between the resources that should be invested in prevention and health promotion activities in order to reduce the number of visits and overall demand for medical care services (demand management) versus those resources that should be spent on taking care of those who require treatment (care management). The second trade-off is between the resources that should be spent on the individual patient versus what should be made available for the anticipated health care needs of all enrollees at large. Managing patient risk broadens and complicates physicians' ethical responsibilities because consideration must be given not only to individual patients but to groups and populations of people who may or may not become patients as well (Shortell, Waters, Clarke, and Budetti, 1998). Having been trained primarily to diagnose and treat sick people, most physicians are uncomfortable making these trade-off decisions. As a result, these decisions are often made by default, frequently with disastrous consequences for patients and physicians alike—both financially and clinically.

To manage risk successfully, partnerships between health systems and physicians must adopt and implement a population-based approach to practicing medicine; another term is "population-based health care management approach." This requires thinking in terms of denominators and not numerators alone and thinking more in terms of maintaining and creating health rather than treating illness. It requires adopting an epidemiological community-based approach to health care delivery. Skills are needed in health status assessment, translation of data into setting priorities for action, implementing prevention and care management systems based on identified priorities, working with others who possess resources and capabilities that extend beyond those of health systems or physicians, and obtaining feedback in order to take corrective action, maintain progress, or set higher targets for achievement. Aligned internal financial incentives are key to making this happen.

### Foundational Properties

Development of these five capabilities is dependent on existence of three characteristics that serve as a foundation.

#### Leadership and Empowerment

Among the biggest challenges in physician integration is creating a common aim or purpose sufficient to get people to work continuously on the relationship to make it succeed. Central to this process is the need to empower physicians, which will require new skills and mind-sets for nonphysician executives.

In a world characterized by increasing paradox (Handy, 1994), perhaps the ultimate paradox in health care is the need to empower physicians. As one of the most dominant groups in the history of the professions (Begun and Lippincott, 1993; Freidson 1970a, 1970b; Light, 1993; Stevens, 1971), how is it that physicians need to be empowered? The answer lies in the recognition that most physicians are at a comparative disadvantage in dealing with the complex financial, managerial, and organizational issues associated with the delivery of health care today. These issues have largely been addressed by a growing cadre of health services executives trained in health services management programs within schools of public health and business management, as well as by executives from other industries who have been recruited into health care.

Historically, there has been a relative separation of medicine and management, with the voluntary medical staff serving as the primary forum for resolving problems and differences. But managed care and related economic, political, and social forces have created a high degree of interdependence of medicine and management, disrupting past relationships. The issues raised by the new relationships are now discussed in economic units involving group practices, IPAs, PHOs, MSOs, equity, and related models that attempt to create incentives for more concerted action. As the transformation of health care increasingly focuses on reorganizing how patient care is delivered, physicians' expertise and experience grow in importance while, paradoxically, their ability to be the sole purveyor of even their clinical autonomy is being eroded. Yet physicians obviously possess important knowledge that nonclinical health care executives do not—regarding what services from a clinical perspective might be offered, regarding treatment alternatives, what clinical outcome measures can be reliably and validly developed, and how new technology is likely to influence treatment patterns and related issues. The separation between administrative and clinical decision making has been largely abolished. The need for greater clinical input combined with physicians' need to continue to exert major control over their work has created the imperative for greater physician empowerment.

Two factors are essential for empowerment to work. First, those being empowered must have the confidence and capability to carry out the tasks delegated to them and be motivated to do so (Rundall,

Starkweather, and Norrish, 1998). It does little good, and, some might argue, much harm, to empower people who are largely unable to execute what they are being empowered to do. In brief, *empowerment* means not only to delegate but to provide with the power (that is training, tools, and so on) to succeed.

Second, for empowerment to work, those in positions of authority and leadership must be willing to let go and share some of their authority with others. This is particularly difficult for those with a high need for control (Bradford and Cohen, 1984) and who have primarily exerted leadership through their formal organization position. It is particularly difficult in health care organizations where considerable distrust has historically existed between executives and physicians (Shortell, 1991; Alexander and others, 1996a). Physicians and health care executives have to earn each other's trust. More physicians have to be prepared to pick up the leadership reins and educate themselves regarding the financial, managerial, and organizational issues associated with modern health care delivery. At the same time, health care executives must learn more about the clinical practice of medicine and understand the important role that leadership plays in improving clinical outcomes of care. Health care executives must also be willing to invest in developing physician leaders and then to share power with them.

Study systems are addressing these issues by working to create a culture that emphasizes collaboration; by investing in systemwide physician education leadership development programs, often jointly with nursing and nonclinical health executives; and by significant growth over the past four years in physician involvement—not only in the management and governance of their own organizations, but also in the larger management and governance of the health system with which they are affiliated. Almost all physician organizations have physician executives as leaders, and most boards of these organizations are dominated by physicians. In many cases, physicians are the lead executives of an overall regional system that comprises several hospitals as well as physician groups. There is some evidence that such involvement is positively associated with higher operating performance (Molinari, Alexander, Morlock, and Lyles, 1995). Increasingly systems are centering their strategic planning process around physician groups rather than hospitals, and in some cases physicians are playing a lead role in implementing overall system mergers. For example, in recent merger discussions involving the Baylor Health System, Harris Methodist, and Presbyterian St. Luke's in the Dallas–Fort Worth marketplace, over one hundred physicians actively participated in all aspects of the discussions. Although the proposed merger was not implemented, everyone agreed that the quality of relationships between and among the different groups of physicians and their respective systems was strengthened by the process. Some other examples of the growing involvement and empowerment of physicians are indicated by the following field notes:

> The extensive involvement of the medical group in the joint strategic planning and management with the system at large is a plus. The involvement is at multiple levels: the system board, top management leadership positions within the system, and key task forces and councils throughout the system.

> The system is open, and visible positioning of physicians in the system helps build legitimacy and trust.

> The system helps to build a portfolio of structures for involving physicians in the system. It helps to develop needed physician resources and skills. Physician leaders are a strong element. Physician leaders are trained and are in key leadership roles. The system focuses on partnership with physicians.

> Leadership development is available and encouraged for those who want it.

The development of the PHO opened up opportunities for physicians to get involved in leadership and governance. The balance of physician to hospital leadership on the board (70 percent physicians and 30 percent others) helps it function as a physician-driven organization.

Equitable representation of primary care physicians on the board of the medical group board helps them feel that they have an effective voice in decision making. For example, primary care physicians are represented in compensation decisions and planning on investments and growth and expansion of the group.

The system has identified desired specific skill sets and leadership competencies in advance. They also emphasize the importance of change management skills and a market orientation. They combine an outside expert with an inside organization development person. This approach could prove useful to others.

### Governance and Management

Improved governance and management of physician organizations and of the relationship between physician organizations and other health care entities (health systems and health plans) is an urgent need. Although improvements have been made over the past four years, many physician organizations are still governed and managed by "popular election" and often with a mind-set of protecting turf and the status quo rather than actively engaging the opportunities for positive change. Fundamentally, physicians and those who work with them need to recognize that medicine is a business as well as a profession. Physician organizations both internally and in their relationship with external groups require more sophisticated governance and management. In particular, the following needs are paramount:

- Recognize the new external reporting and account-ability demands and learn to participate in a system of shared mutual accountability with private and public sector organizations, or accrediting bodies, and related groups.

- Learn to govern and manage the increasing size of medical groups, particularly in dealing with issues of diseconomies of scale and scope, attenuation of incentives that come with size, increasing bureaucracy, and related issues (Robinson, 1999b).

- Clearly spell out roles and responsibilities at all levels of governance and management within the physician group and in relationships with outside parties.

The following examples from the field notes illustrate these points:

Organizational mentoring, whereby a new clinic is linked with a successful clinic, has been used to teach other clinics successful techniques. New clinics being brought on board understand from the beginning that they will be required to use a common information system.

The Integrated Products Council is an innovative approach to arriving at a conceptual decision-making framework regarding single-signature contracting and related issues. This council is made of up six members from the system and six from the medical group. But there are only two votes, such that each group must come to full consensus and agreement in casting their group vote, and action is not taken unless both groups are in agreement.

The design of the group in terms of the primary care–specialty physician relationship is based on an open access model. This has prevented a lot of potential conflict. Also, effort is made to maintain a balance of primary care physicians and specialists on all committees, and this helped to address a potential conflicting relationship.

The extensive representation of community representatives on the physician group board is innovative. Not only does this tie the group to the community, but it also perhaps mitigates unnecessary conflict that could arise if more of the board members came from the system at large. The community members offer a different perspective and help to eliminate some of the otherwise inherent conflict that might exist between physicians and hospital executives.

The physician division regional medical director is a key position for physician-system alignment. The position is both clinical and administrative. These directors serve on the health system board and provide feedback to their division. They also oversee cost measures (relative value units) and quality and satisfaction measures. They are an important link to help build strong relationships between the system and the rank-and-file physicians.

The joint management and planning organization allows for joint planning and contracting between the hospital and independent physicians. This facilitates the development of an employed physicians' group by lessening the concerns of the independent physicians. There is joint physician manpower planning, with the right of first refusal on the part of the independent physicians.

*Capital*

The robust properties previously discussed require ongoing capital investment even though some of the individual properties themselves (leadership development programs, for example) are not necessarily capital intensive The big-ticket item, of course, is the investment in information technology and, beyond that, the capital required to purchase physician practices to the extent that this makes sense. The experiences of the study systems to date suggest that these investments need to be considered within the context of the whole, that is, the other robust properties identified. Without an emphasis and understanding of denominator-based population-based medicine, aligned financial incentives, a commitment to CQI, trustworthy leadership, and effective governance and management, the capital investment in information technology or the further purchase of physician practices is unlikely to be leveraged. Just as some systems have pulled out of the health plan business so they could better deploy their capital elsewhere, some systems may want to go more slowly in their investment in information technology or continued acquisition of physician practices and redirect some of the capital to expanding CQI efforts using existing information or investing in existing physician practices. Some systems have already placed strict limits on the amount of capital they will invest per new physician acquired. For example, one of the study systems limits this figure at $100,000 per physician.

## Future Issues

The medical profession is going through a painful period where nearly everything is changing at once. All of the pillars and handrails of the pier have been torpedoed, and there is nothing left to grab onto. Based on our most recent research and field experience, we suggest that the best thing for both physicians and health systems executives to do is to just let go. The pier needs to be rebuilt altogether, and we have proposed eight pillars—the robust properties—that we believe will provide a firm foundation for the future.

Fundamental changes in physician-system integration relationships have not yet resulted from increased managed care pressures (Morrisey, Alexander, Burns, and Johnson, 1999). This reflects the fact that most efforts at physician integration over the past four years have been largely defensive, designed to protect past economic relationships and preserve the status quo. This is understandable. But it is now time to move forward. Galvin (1998) has asked the central question: "Can physicians form organizations that challenge doctors to look at the bigger picture than just their immediate professional needs and excite them about working in teams to improve quality and face the issue of restructuring?"

Of the available options, relatively few organizations will be able to be successful starting from scratch. The Mayo, Geisinger, Cleveland, Ochsner, Scott-White, Carle, Lahey, Marshfield, and Virginia Mason Clinics of the world have very different organizational markings and genetics than do the start-up physician organizations of today. Today's physician organizations largely lack the capital and managerial and organizational expertise to go it alone and, in particular, are not good at managing growth.

The failure of the physician practice management (PPM) option has largely embarrassed investors and industry observers alike who felt that the PPMs could be a viable source of capital for the growth of effective physician practices (Burns and Robinson, 1997). Although a second generation of PPMs may be better able to target niche markets, the PPM strategy is not likely to be a viable option for most physicians or medical groups. It is also not clear that health plans want to be in the physician management business or have any comparative advantage in doing so.

This leaves hospitals and health systems as the residual partner. In many cases, physicians have been alienated and driven off by what they perceive (rightly or wrongly) as efforts by hospitals and health systems to control the delivery system with little input from physicians. This has now began to change, and the climate for more fruitful system-physician integration is better today in most places than it was four years ago. In fact, some systems are striking partnerships with physician groups on the rebound from negative experience with PPMs. For example, Cardinal Healthcare has reached an agreement with three hospitals in North Carolina's Triangle region allowing the eighty-member physician group to buy itself back from its troubled partner, Med Partners. Cardinal, which has about 200,000 patients, will sell a minority partnership to UNC Healthcare, Wake Med, and Rex Healthcare, which in turn will lend Cardinal "millions of dollars." The investment banker in this arrangement noted, "You could certainly look at [the three hospitals] as the white knights riding in on the white horses" (*Internet News*, 1999).

Based on a current assessment of the evolving experience of the study systems, we foresee continued experimentation with different physician integration strategies. Whether the specific models will be tight or loose, physicians will need to be part of an organizational process that supports the delivery of coordinated care to patients in need and disease prevention and health promotion services to those who are well. Following are some suggestions for increasing the probability that these partnerships will work:

- Focus effort and attention on the patient.

- Make quality of health care the overarching goal of all partners, a goal that everyone can buy into.

- Develop and maintain a culture that gives priority to sharing information and improving the ability to meet patient needs.

- Provide opportunities for partners to work together on meaningful issues and actively promote teamwork.

Side issues or past conflicts should not prevent forward movement on core issues facing the partnership today.

- Actively promote mutual understanding of the short-term needs and interests of all partners. People will not see the long term if certain short-term needs are not recognized.

- Maintain a balance between short-term and long-term needs of all partners, and show how achieving short-term objectives will promote meeting long-term needs.

- Foster leadership skills among all partners; partners should be committed to the recruitment and retention of those with such skills.

- Identify specific barriers to the partnership; all concerned members should work together to eliminate these barriers.

- Recognize the potential for new structures and multiple structures in order to support the needs of all parties. Be flexible; the means should serve the ends.

- Evaluate and monitor the different models to determine what works best and spread the lessons learned to other relationships. This will require developing explicit objectives and performance measures for the relationship.

These suggestions are consistent with the "I" principles of effective partnerships based on experience in other sectors: importance, investment, interdependence, integrated, informed, institutionalized, and integrity (Kanter, 1994). Everything should be done to ensure that the relationship between the system and physicians is seen as important to each party. For example, as consolidation continues among health plans, it will become increasingly important for providers to consolidate as well. This will provide an incentive for both hospital and health systems and physicians to join together and for physicians to consolidate into larger economic groups while attempting to maintain a small enough scale of practice to deliver personalized care. The importance of larger size will move from the ability to secure managed care contracts to developing the ability to manage patient care risk in order to perform successfully under these contracts.

From an investment perspective, both hospitals and health systems and physicians need to mature as business partners in working with each other. While working to achieve short-run objectives, each needs to recognize the long-run objectives of the relationship. Decision making on the part of all parties needs to be based not only on a mutual set of shared values but also on principles of good business decision making. What may make sense for physicians at one point in time will not for hospitals or health systems, and vice versa. Yet each needs to recognize the legitimate business interests of the other party.

Everything should be done to increase the interdependence between physicians and the hospital and health system. This interdependence will broaden to include payers and consumer groups in regard to mutual accountability (Gosfield, 1998; Shortell, Waters, Clarke and Budetti, 1998). Physicians and physician organizations will need the capital of hospitals and health systems to provide needed information for purposes of external reporting as well as for purposes of internal continuous improvement. These needs will heighten the interdependency of these parties.

The relationship between hospital and health systems and physicians must become increasingly integrated through aligned financial incentives and shared decision making. Formal organized processes for shared decision making must be implemented. Gosfield (1998) suggests four categories of physician involvement:

- Decisions in which it is *imperative* for physicians to be involved—for example, selection of new physicians into a practice, development and implementation of care management practices, determination of compensation and financial incentives, and implementation of CQI initiatives

- Decisions for which it will be *very important* for physician involvement—for example, information systems development, risk management strategies, and strategic planning

- Decisions for which it will be *useful* for physicians to be involved—for example, financial reporting systems and marketing

- Decisions that are *not a priority* for physician involvement but might on occasion be useful—for example, nonclinical support services decisions and public relations

The relationship between hospital and health systems and physicians must be as fully informed as possible. The technical aspects of information systems must be married with decision-making structures that can effectively use the information. This is related to the shared decision-making examples associated with effective management and governance.

The relationship needs to become increasingly institutionalized in regard to daily practice. This is needed to develop an infrastructure of trust that extends through daily decision making and the governance and management structures of the organizations, and is recognized in the implementation of the robust properties discussed in this chapter.

Finally, the relationship must be based on integrity. This is characterized by following through on what one says one is going to do, being open and honest in communication, and being willing to help each other develop further capabilities to achieve mutual goals.

Our examination of the evidence and experience to date suggests that it is the relationships that matter most, not the specific models. The ultimate test of physician-system integration efforts will be the extent to which they lead to more effective coordination of services to patients and populations so as to create greater value for consumers and purchasers.

### Sentara Healthcare

Sentara Healthcare, headquartered in Norfolk, Virginia, has eighteen physicians in management positions throughout the system. It was not always that way. The push to include physicians in management started in August 1994 with the creation of a single board for Sentara and the formation of the Executive Council with a composition of 50 percent physicians and 50 percent management. This was a watershed event. Today physicians at Sentara work in a variety of positions, including the chief medical officer of the system, medical directors for the hospitals, medical director for Sentara health management, vice president for medical affairs, vice president for medical management, medical director of clinical effectiveness, executive medical director of the medical group, senior medical director of the health plan, vice president of the physician network, and medical directors for product lines such as cardiology and oncology. In addition to these full-time employed physicians, other physicians affiliated with Sentara participate on the health system board and leadership councils.

### Progress Toward Physician Integration

Sentara's 1999–2003 strategic plan recounts the three phases that have characterized physician integration over the past two decades through the first decade of the new century.

The first phase in the 1980s, when Sentara began to create the different component parts of a system, was to align the interests of hospitals, doctors, and clinics. It was not yet an integrated delivery system, although there was extensive discussion of the benefits that integration would yield. From the beginning, this discussion included participation from each of their three components: care delivery (hospitals, outpatient and long-term care), physicians, and health plans.

During the 1990s the focus in the second phase shifted to greater emphasis on the health plan and managing patient care. With enactment of the federal Health Security Act of 1993, Sentara adopted a strong growth strategy that included an imperative to increase the number of "covered lives." Sentara developed clinical benchmarks and began to look in depth at medical management. Organizationally, it developed a spectrum of relationship models, including MSO-type services up to and including an employment model. Sentara currently employs over 160 physicians, approximately 90 percent of whom are primary care providers. An IPA was formed but no longer exists; however, other relationships and "virtual" (non-employed) models have evolved.

The evolution in the third phase, now in process, is catalyzed by a strategic decision to focus on the patient. Sentara believes it must provide a consumer-based health system emphasizing the quality of care if it is to be successful in the coming decade. Physicians must be involved in this strategy in ways that allow a customized fit with the organization for the providers while maintaining attention to patient needs.

## Keys to Success

There are several keys to success in the way that Sentara has strategically managed physician integration. One important decision was to develop a central chief medical officer position in 1995. This person has responsibilities for improving clinical quality and reducing costs within the hospitals and through the health plan. He also works to further physician relationships, meet and exceed clinical benchmarks, and provide leadership to physicians and the medical staff.

From a statutory perspective, the abandonment of a corporate practice of medicine act in Virginia in 1993 was helpful in operationalizing cooperation. Some physicians had already realized at that time that there was a "hang together or hang separately" reality to their situation. And this hanging together needed to be with the health system, not just with other physicians. These physicians identified benefits to working together with the health system. This collaboration focused on access to medical care for patients, recruiting and retaining primary care physicians, and incorporating physician leadership councils in management processes.

Another key to success in physician integration at Sentara is the development of a common understanding of the external environment and what it takes organizationally to survive in that environment. One of the principal vehicles for securing this shared understanding is the clinical college, also known as the Health Management Forum. The forum is an attempt to use educational materials to help Sentara-affiliated physicians understand the demands and requirements of managed care from both a clinical and a managerial point of view. Designed by a physician affiliated with Sentara and others associated with the Graduate School of Business at the College of William and Mary, the program has provided seminars in business and clinical care effectiveness to over 230 physicians. The business classes, limited in size to 45 members, emphasize cost accounting and cost reduction in medical practice, informatics in medical practice, measuring clinical outcomes in medical practice, marketing physician services, and negotiation strategies. The clinical care effectiveness classes have grown in enrollment in each of the three years they have been in place, from 85 physicians in the first year to over 120 in the most recent year. The seminars are provided at no cost to the physician participants. The total cost of the program is less than $250,000 per year.

Among the tools used at the forum are case studies such as "Paragon Healthcare," developed by Sentara physicians and professors in the Graduate School of Business at the College of William and Mary. This case study emphasizes the requirements of responding to a request for proposal to participate in a specialty care network (gastroenterology) and convert from fee for service to capitation. In the beginning, Sentara conducted physician focus groups to assess their interests and maintain close communication on physician preferences for topics. There are some research and development activities taking place regarding this program. For example, a Web-based version of a monograph is being developed. Another example is the information system and electronic medical record effort underway at Sentara. Program management believes that there is a teaching opportunity to work on this development at least in part in a classroom setting.

The forum educational program has become a new way to communicate with physicians and will likely be even more important in the future. On the clinical side, program development often starts with asking a question, such as, "How much are we spending in the Sentara system on a specific clinical service such as asthma care?" Someone at Sentara had noticed that they had too many emergency room visits and too many hospitalizations in their system of people with asthma. They created a task force of managers and physicians who met and developed a monograph that was used in a clinical seminar, implemented in clinical practice in some locations, and followed up using the data system to see if there were demonstrable changes in clinical practices. Information from the data system is compared with standards from Milliman and Roberts (a data management benchmarking company) to discern opportunities for further improvement. In general their process is to develop an algorithm and monograph and limit these efforts to a maximum of five to six clinical targets each year.

On the health plan side, 50 percent of the board of directors of the health plan are physicians. Sentara has developed specialty advisory councils for six to eight specialties with six to ten physicians from each specialty working on a council. The advisory councils help the health plan in addressing clinical issues, implementing protocols, and developing medical management benchmarks (for the specialist's specialty). Plans are being discussed to have these advisory councils evolve into a virtual multispecialty group of key physicians in the community and develop a focused point-of-service product with these physicians' participation.

A final key to success involves responding to physicians' issues and needs. For example, physicians requested information about their practice patterns because comparative information was beginning to be made public. Sentara responded with the Physician Report Portfolio. In its third version in approximately one year, the portfolio provides information that is available from the state, national sources, Sentara hospitals, and Sentara's health plan for a physician's practice. Clinicians are provided detailed reports on severity-adjusted length of stay and charge comparisons among peers within a hospital, severity-adjusted data on a large number of clinical, financial, and quality outcome measurements, and other reports from the health plan.

## Obstacles and Barriers to Physician Integration

One of the key barriers to physician integration is ambivalence on the part of some physicians regarding being part of a big company. Some physicians are afraid to trust or depend too much on any one health care organization. There is a perception that perhaps younger physicians may be different in this regard compared to older, more established physicians—that is, younger physicians may have different expectations on such matters as group practice, managed care, integrated systems, and salaries, along with different perceptions of their work. Older physicians often have had more robust expectations and are looking to retire rather than deal with changes they do not like. Many older physicians also feel that the profession suffers from lower public esteem than it enjoyed in the past. Although younger physicians may be more accepting of the new challenges in the profession, they may not be willing to spend as many hours in clinical work as physicians did ten to fifteen years ago. Lifestyle issues affect the balance of work and other demands on their time. For example, call coverage for trauma and other increasing demands on physicians' time pose challenges.

Another challenge has been the organizational configurations of the physicians in medical groups. With the merger of the Sentara and Tidewater health systems in 1998, there were a number of elements that needed to be harmonized. For example, each system had a large primary care practice that was principally affiliated with that specific system, and these groups were affiliated with historically rival systems. As part of the overall merger agreement, it was determined that the two medical groups would merge over three years. During this time, they would collaborate on how to merge the two groups and evolve structures, policies, and payment schemes. Early meetings yielded a surprising willingness to work together. Physician representatives from both medical groups, the president, and the chief medical officer of Sentara began meetings in August 1999, and thus far the pace is much faster than anticipated. Progress toward full integration appears to be accelerated and motivated at least in part by the desire of the physicians in the group to move away from uncertainty toward certainty.

## Lessons Learned

One of the key lessons for Sentara is that the system found that maintaining a separate hospital staff structure was not helpful for its goals. Rather, physicians need to be incorporated into the organization so that they may be involved throughout the whole decision-making process. Sentara has brought eighteen physicians into key management positions, and this experience has been very positive. The new responsibilities have given the physicians a perspective they did not have before. Typically, once the physicians have been in these positions for a year or two, they develop a greater understanding of the system and system requirements as a whole, and they make important contributions to management. Physicians who are operating well within the system lend credence to the system with other physicians and help explain the logic of actions taken.

Sentara has found that the opportunities for physician involvement vary. Some physicians are permanently placed in management, and some are on physicians' councils, which look at issues of cost, quality, and the use of clinical protocols. For example, Sentara has two councils of twelve physicians each based on market area, with these members primarily practicing physicians. Physicians are also members of Sentara's three key management committees (strategy, medical management, and operations management).

Managers at Sentara have learned the importance of being "physician friendly" in order to improve operations, including operation of the health plan. Many of the physicians had been annoyed with HMOs in general, and the Sentara health plan was no exception. Management talked with the senior physicians who constituted the "peerage of the medical staff." These physicians indicated that there should be an intrinsic value in the Sentara system's having its own HMO and that the HMO should be responsive to system physicians. In fact, one of Sentara's strengths is that the senior medical director of medical management of the HMO is a local physician who is very available to Sentara physicians and patients.

◆　◆　◆　◆　◆　◆

## Future Directions

The future appears to hold an opportunity for more integration and collaboration with physicians. Although there is already preliminary activity in the area of setting up collaborative ambulatory surgery centers, complementary and alternative medicine services, outpatient ancillary services, and health and fitness centers, for example, even more of this activity will be catalyzed if the certificate-of-need law in Virginia is eliminated as expected. Currently there are three pilot programs in alternative medicine underway built on ideas initiated by the physicians. In addition, the "virtual" specialty group product will continue to be developed and implemented during the next year as the Sentara Health Plan works to reorganize itself to meet the needs of its physician and patient members. Future challenges and opportunities involve working with the medical group physicians to develop a new successor group, establish "soft landings" for physicians who opt out of the successor group, and develop "virtual" physician models to maintain strong relationships with physicians. In addition, efforts to improve cost and quality of care through clinical and management teams will continue.

## Fairview Physician Associates

When we profiled Fairview's physician system integration strategy in 1995, we focused on Fairview Physician Associates, the system physician organization created by Fairview and medical staff leaders from its Twin Cities hospitals. FPA was born out of necessity. In the early 1990s, a large employer coalition was formed with intentions to contract more directly with an exclusive provider group. The Buyers Health Care Action Group (BHCAG), as the coalition is now referred to, did not select Fairview and its loosely defined physician contracting entity. This set off an early-warning alarm for Fairview physician and administrative leadership and created a substantial zone of discomfort for the existing physician system organizational structure.

As was the case with many of the regional systems in the Health Systems Integration Study, Fairview and its physicians were also anticipating the impact of health reform at the state and national levels. The Minnesota legislature had enacted Minnesota Care; the most significant cost containment and organizational changes in this plan for state health reform called for health care to be purchased through integrated service networks (ISNs). The early definition of ISNs indicated that they were to be "organizations accountable for the costs and outcomes associated with delivering a full continuum of services to a defined population." The legislature had recognized the need to reform a "fragmented non-system of independent providers," many of whom were paid on a piecemeal basis, "into coordinated networks capable of providing all care for a fixed price."

Our initial case study of FPA addressed the visioning of the organization, its original board and management structure, and its unique way of handling physicians who desired to have differing levels of commitment to FPA and those physician groups providing care at Fairview facilities and at competing facilities. We described an organization that wanted to create a "fee-for-quality" compensation methodology for its members, whereby physicians would be paid more or less depending on how well they performed relative to key measures developed by FPA. We also indicated that the BHCAG had become frustrated with its initial choice of an exclusive network and was looking to redesign its strategy to include other primary care–based systems in a new offering to its members and their employees.

## Progress Toward Integration

Although FPA's initial formation years can be described as a time of visioning, creating, and establishing, the years covered by our current case study are best described as a period of implementing, actualizing, achieving, and maturing. The annual reports of FPA and FPA's membership meetings highlight a growing set of accomplishments. Some focus on achieving greater integration of care management, and many reveal an organization that has clearly moved beyond its early roots as a contracting network.

The development of a fee-for-quality compensation methodology is becoming a reality. Quality and care management are the drivers of the payment model, which includes four key elements:

- System reward pool. The system reward pool is funded by a commitment of the Fairview system to contribute 5 percent of the payments received by Fairview hospitals and the rest of the continuum of care providers. These funds can be distributed according to the attainment of system performance objectives. Past objectives include patient satisfaction, the amount of care provided within the FPA care system, implementation of a depression management guideline, and pharmaceutical management.

- Physician performance. This component of the compensation methodology encourages FPA providers to actively participate in and increase their understanding of FPA's initiatives. The importance of addressing the physician performance goals is well understood by FPA's members. Goals must be achieved before there is a payout of surplus, and attaining the objectives also helps a clinic avoid a future withhold on reimbursement. As with the system performance objectives, the specific physician per-formance objectives will change from year to year to address be-havior changes and quality improvement opportunities. Among past objectives are participation in FPA's patient and provider sat-isfaction survey process, completion of a clinic-based quality-improvement initiative, and participation in ongoing clinic site leader and administrative forums.

- Risk fund withhold. In recent years, FPA's Product Development and Contracting Committee has set the withhold amount to be 3 percent of fee schedule payments.

- FPA fees schedule. FPA has developed its own internal fee schedule through which to distribute the capitation payments re-ceived from payers.

The adoption and implementation of the compensation model has helped tie the financial incentives of membership participation to the strategies and care management goals of the organization.

Although FPA was initially formed in response to not being awarded a provider contract by the BHCAG, in 1996 the group struc-tured a new "care system" approach to contracting with providers. To qualify as a care system, a provider must be a primary care cen-tered health system with its affiliated specialty hospital and allied pro-fessional arrangements that offers either directly or through contracts with other organizations the full continuum of medically necessary services for an enrolled population. The structure and strategy of FPA met this definition for the BHCAG, and in a competitive RFP process FPA became one of the care systems selected by the action group to serve its employees and their families. This selection rewarded the work efforts and sweat equity contributed by many of FPA's founders. It also helped propel the covered lives under management by FPA providers to a critical mass of sixty thousand.

FPA's integration efforts have not stopped with the traditional functions designed to make an IPA function effectively. In pursuing its vision of creating an integrated provider network, FPA implemented an electronic medical record (EMR) pilot program in 1999. The inauguration of an EMR was seen as a means to help a member clinic work more effectively across all aspects of its operations, not just the activities or patients covered by an FPA-managed care contract. For FPA, the implementation of the EMR has helped to fulfill many of its physician leaders' dreams for a computer system that easily schedules appointments, updates patient records, orders prescription drugs, and generates bills.

## Obstacles and Barriers to Integration

As is true for most systems in the Health Systems Integration Study, the late 1990s have been characterized by system strategies focused on cost cutting in order to stay within the payment reductions being extracted by Medicare through implementation of the Balanced Budget Act. Fairview has been forced to scale back on some capital deployment in response to reduced operating margins. This has been a factor in the implementation of FPA's strategy. In the spring of 1996, FPA announced that it was within "spitting distance" of selecting its patient-focused EMR system. The piloting of the program, however, took three years to materialize, in part because of the capital crunch within the Fairview system.

A second barrier to FPA's ongoing integration efforts is the implementation of strategy and structures for physicians who are in very different practice organizational and ownership structures. A substantial portion of FPA's primary care physicians (PCPs) are employed by Fairview, but FPA's independent PCPs are also major players in the provision of and access to primary care offered by FPA. Many independent primary care physicians and independent specialists have been long-term supporters of Fairview and contributors to the system's success. The Twin Cities environment is characterized by the formation of large single-specialty group practices that provide care at many hospitals and systems, some of which compete with Fairview. This prevents them from concentrating their efforts purely on FPA providers, and it has at times made them fearful about committing to FPA out of concern for the non-FPA primary care physicians who refer patients to them.

A third obstacle for FPA has been Fairview's acquisition of the University of Minnesota Hospital and the need to integrate its activities within Fairview and to establish relationships with the university-employed faculty physicians. The sheer size and complexity of this academic community health system has consumed management time and resources that five years ago were being dedicated to making FPA successful.

## Keys to Success

At its core, eight years after the formation of its initial vision statement FPA remains committed to the attainment of that vision. The organization prides itself on regular written and electronic communication. FPA regularly brings its membership together in educational forums, membership meetings, and meaningful committee work.

Clinic administrators have been included in decision making and committee leadership since day one of FPA's organization. The involvement of the clinic administrators has helped foster communication and create effective linkages for the implementation of FPA's strategies.

Unlike many physician organizations, once patients or members elect the FPA system for their care they are typically not required to get a referral from a primary care physician to see a specialist within the FPA network. This helps underscore the overall quality of the network and the trust relationship that continues to develop between primary care physicians and specialists. FPA does maintain a referral office, but its purpose is not to authorize or question referrals. Instead, this system offers feedback to the members of FPA on the physicians who are receiving referrals for specialty care. It also provides an important assessment on the amount of care that is being given within versus outside of the FPA network.

## Lessons Learned

FPA leaders can share countless stories of the tuition they paid in the school of hard knocks that one goes through in creating and implementing a physician system organization. Three lessons are particularly noteworthy. The first is consistency in dedicated leadership. FPA's paid physician president and vice president of operations have been with the organization from its formation. This continuity has fostered a stable culture while everything else in the environment is changing. It also has facilitated the recruitment of excellent staff and created a working relationship with other leaders in the Fairview system that is characterized by problem solving versus ongoing problem identification.

A second important lesson is the importance of securing a book of business. When FPA began to negotiate and sign contacts with one of the Twin Cities' major managed care companies and with the BHCAG, FPA's members began to take the organization seriously. A critical mass of covered lives is essential in order for providers and their clinic administrators to commit the resources necessary to make a physician network successful.

A third lesson learned from FPA is the importance of addressing the needs of independent primary care physicians, specialty groups, and employed system physicians in the governance, operation, and resource allocation of and for the physician organization. When FPA implemented the pilot site for its electronic medical record, the clinic selected was one owned and operated by an independent primary care practice. The emphasis could have been placed on an owned Fairview clinic and employed physicians, but FPA leadership recognized the need to establish principles of fairness in resource allocation decisions.

## Future Challenges

FPA has matured to the point where its dedicated infrastructure is able to assist its physicians in the effective management and delivery of care. The challenge for the future is to continue to demonstrate value to its members and to purchasers in order to grow the base of covered lives under management by FPA. A critical mass of covered lives has been achieved by FPA, but continued growth will assist FPA in the battle for more capital resources. FPA's current strategy is oriented toward this goal, with a dual focus on enhanced care management and the continued improvement in patient and provider satisfaction with the FPA network. In the months and years ahead, the piloting of the EMR will be closely tracked to evaluate its ability to improve care delivery, practice operations, and patient satisfaction. As the integration of the University of Minnesota hospital into Fairview continues, FPA can anticipate initiatives to explore substantive relationships between FPA and the University of Minnesota faculty physicians.

# 5

. . . . . . . . . . . . . . . . . . . . . . . . . . . . . . . . . . . . . . .

# Clinical Integration

Clinical integration is the extent to which patient care services are coordinated across people, functions, activities, and sites over time so as to maximize the value of services delivered to patients. We continue to believe that it is the most important element in the ability of organized delivery systems to achieve more cost-effective delivery of care because it is most directly associated with the provision of such care. This chapter presents new evidence and observations on clinical integration based on the experiences of the study systems over the past four years, assessment of the experiences of selected other systems, and a review of current literature.

In 1996, the study systems were only beginning to work on clinical integration, having focused most of their attention and energy in the early 1990s on putting the pieces of the system together, building a functional infrastructure, and negotiating relationships with physicians. We found low to modest perceived levels of clinical integration—2.5 on a 1 to 5 (low to high) scale in both 1991 and 1992—and this had actually decreased slightly to 2.4 in 1994. The two factors most strongly related to a greater degree of clinical integration were standardization of information systems and various measures of physician system integration. In particular, the greater was the percentage of physicians practicing in groups (particularly groups of twenty-five physicians or more), the greater was the degree of shared clinical service lines, shared clinical support services, and shared medical records. Also, the greater the degree of physician involvement in management there was, the more likely an individual hospital was to share clinical service lines, clinical support services, medical records, clinical outcomes, and protocols.

We also identified a number of barriers and challenges to clinical integration organized under four dimensions that we labeled strategic, structural, cultural, and technical. As a whole, these barriers and challenges included the following factors:

- Lack of a specific strategy and implementation plan for achieving clinical integration

- Lack of or misalignment of internal incentives to achieve clinical integration

- Too few physician groups

- Dispersed geography

- The institutional autonomy of hospitals

- Employee fears of job loss and physician fears of autonomy loss

- Inadequate information systems

Based on our new round of interviews with the top management leadership of each system and an examination of existing documents, it is clear that these barriers largely remain today. In addition, we would add a new barrier: a relative lack of focus on clinical integration priorities due to disruptive external financial demands related to the Balanced Budget Amendment Act of 1997 and concern regarding Y2K information system compliance. As one respondent noted, "Focusing on clinical integration is fine when the organization is in a steady state. But it's very difficult to do clinical integration work when a gun is being held to your head."

## Recent Update

As with physician integration, we collected information from the top management teams on twelve clinical integration activities:

- Development and implementation of clinical guidelines, protocols, and pathways

- Implementation of a common patient identifier

- Use of case management systems

- Disease management systems

- Demand management systems

- Implementation of population-based community health models

- Implementation of clinical information systems

- Use of inpatient CQI

- Use of outpatient and primary care–oriented CQI

- Use of inpatient clinical service lines

- Use of both inpatient and outpatient clinical service lines

- Quality improvement steering councils

Most systems were involved in each of these activities, except for demand management programs, which were used by only two of the study systems. Information was collected on the levels at which decisions were made (individual operating unit versus shared between the operating unit and region/system versus made at the region/system level); satisfaction with progress (1 = no satisfaction to 5 = very satisfied); importance for achieving integration (1 = not important to 3 = very important); and extent of implementation (1 = not implemented to 3 = fully implemented).

Across all activities and systems, the level of decision making was evenly mixed between centralized and decentralized approaches. The most decentralized activities involved the implementation of a common patient identifier, implementation of inpatient and outpatient CQI, and the implementation of inpatient clinical service lines. The decentralization of CQI activities is a relative change from four years ago when these activities tended to be more centralized at a regional or system level. Based on interviews, this reflects the fact that CQI activity is now being implemented in delivery settings with responsibility and accountability placed at the operating unit level. The only activity of the twelve that was consistently centralized by all systems was the quality steering council. Again, based on interviews, these councils served as an evaluating and monitoring body for all quality improvement activities within the system and also served to facilitate learning and the sharing of best practices across system operating units. All of the remaining activities, from the implementation of guidelines and protocols to clinical information systems, tended to reflect the mixture of centralized and decentralized decision making.

The overall level of satisfaction with the twelve activities was 2.85 on the 5.0 scale, reflecting at best moderate satisfaction with clinical integration to date. The highest satisfaction score was expressed for inpatient CQI implementation, at 3.2, and the lowest for implementation of a common patient identifier, at 2.3.

Almost all of the activities were seen as important, with an overall average of 2.71 on the three-point scale. Clinical information systems and the implementation of outpatient and primary care CQI received the highest importance scores, while the lowest was population-based community health improvement, at 2.2. Interviews revealed that population-based community health improvement was seen as an important overall system objective but more of an overarching goal than a means of achieving clinical integration itself.

The overall average implementation score was 2.7 on the three-point scale. The highest implementation reading was for the common patient identifier, at 2.9, indicating that although few have done this, once a system decides to do it, it either implements it or not. The lowest implementation scores were for the CQI steering council, CQI inpatient implementation, and case management. Again, interviews revealed numerous barriers to implementing these activities.

Clinical integration efforts among the study systems are in a state of flux and experimentation with regard to roles and responsibilities, decision-making levels, and accountability. Although a fair number of initiatives are on the way to implementation, top management respondents are only marginally satisfied with the results produced to date.

Since 1996, systems have grown in their understanding of the demands of clinical integration and have obtained more sophisticated insight into the different levels and processes involved to coordinate patient care better. In the sections that follow, we highlight some new ways of thinking about clinical integration, identify some key success factors, highlight a number of examples illustrating these success factors, and elaborate on future challenges, particularly in regard to the management of multiple chronic illnesses.

## Clinical Integration: Deeper Understanding

Clinical integration is embedded in relationships at three levels. At the most abstract level, clinical integration is embedded within the nature of the financial and legal transactions of the system involving the building blocks of the system. These are corporate-level decisions involving the relationships between and among delivery units such as hospitals, long-term care facilities, and home health agencies; physician practice organizations; and health plans. These vary in important ways in regard to number, size, geographic dispersion, and whether they are owned or contracted. These relationships set the initial boundary conditions within which clinical integration occurs. An organized delivery system that has gaps in the continuum of care of its facilities cannot achieve full integration of care for its population. Similarly, an organized delivery system whose service sites are geographically dispersed will be challenged to provide coordinated care to various segments of its population.

At the intermediate level or managerial level are decisions involving economies of scope and scale; that is, what services will be located at what sites? These decisions involve consolidation, duplication, and potential trade-offs regarding access, cost, and quality. These decisions directly affect clinical integration by placing boundaries on program design. For example, the decision to centralize certain programs or services at a single site means that some patients will need to go to that site to receive the service. This represents a potential discontinuity in care and places a demand on the system's coordination capabilities. Primary among these capabilities are its willingness and ability to standardize care to eliminate unnecessary variation and to foster accurate and timely communication between and among the patient and the patient's caregiver through electronic and face-to-face communication.

The third level involves the technical core within which patient care delivery occurs. This technical core involves both the overall organization of work and the specific processes used to carry out the work. Examples of the overall organization of work include the use of service line management, program management, centers of excellence, and related approaches. Examples of specific processes used to carry out the work include use of clinical guidelines, protocols, pathways, case and care management systems, and disease management approaches. These processes are heavily influenced by the overall organization of work. For example, it is possible to implement a clinical guideline for diabetes in a service line even though the service line may not have budgetary authority. But it is very difficult or impossible to implement a comprehensive care management approach to diabetes care where the service line does not have such authority.

Figure 5.1 shows the three levels of embedded relationships. The importance of understanding these three levels is to recognize the opportunities and constraints that they place on achieving clinical integration. Without this understanding, there is a disconnect between the front-office decision makers and the front-line caregivers that cannot be reconciled. This is one of the fundamental lessons of the study systems' experience over the past four years and, we believe, of the health sector at large. The situation is well summarized by the following statement:

> Though we have seen many health care organizations going about consolidating their assets through mergers and affiliations, we know that this is not true integration. Integration as a *service delivery method* and as an *approach to care* has not been widely tested in mainstream health care. Integration is about bringing together the set of people (health care professionals, social service staff) who serve the same client, either concurrently or at different points in time in different service sectors [Bringewatt, 1999].

In addition to understanding embeddedness, it is important to recognize the notion of interdependence and its implications for integration. In any work process, three basic types of interdependence exist: pooled, sequential, and reciprocal (Thompson, 1967).

Pooled interdependence exists when two or more work processes do not need to interact directly with each other to produce a good or service. Their activities do not need to be directly coordinated; rather, they are coordinated or "pooled" at a higher level in the organization. For example, in putting together a packaged pricing disease management program for cardiovascular care, the marketing and financial staffs do not directly interact with the cardiovascular surgeons; rather, they assemble data on volume and type of surgeries,

Figure 5.1. Embedded Relationships of Clinical Integration.

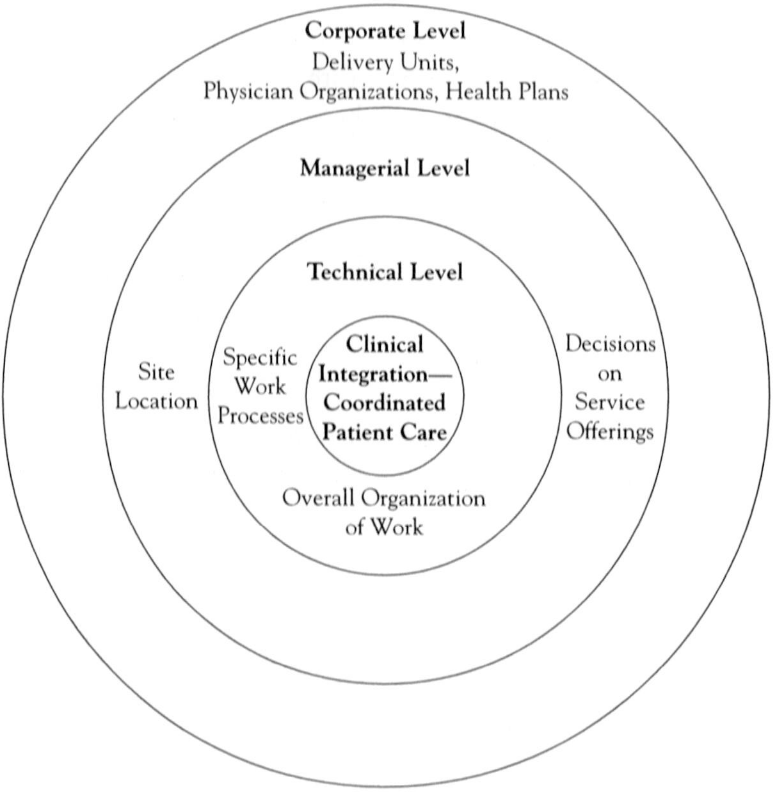

Corporate Level
Delivery Units,
Physician Organizations, Health Plans

Managerial Level

Technical Level

Clinical
Integration—
Coordinated
Patient Care

Specific
Work
Processes

Site
Location

Decisions
on
Service
Offerings

Overall Organization
of Work

costs, outcomes of care, and related information to put together a packaged program.

*Sequential* integration exists when one or more work processes or units is dependent on another to get its work done, but the former does not depend on the latter. This is the classic manufacturing assembly line arrangement. The relationships between and among the operating room, intensive care unit (ICU), step-down unit, and patient floors of a hospital are largely of a sequential nature. The ICU depends on the operating room for the arrival time of the patient, the immediate outcome of the surgery, and instructions for postoperative monitoring and treatment. The operating room is not generally dependent on the ICU. In similar fashion, the step-down unit is dependent on the ICU for pertinent information regarding the transfer of the patient to the step-down unit, but the ICU is essentially not dependent on the step-down unit. In turn, the patient floor is dependent on the step-down unit but not vice versa. When interdependence is primarily of a sequential nature, integration can largely be achieved through the use of written rules, protocols, and instructions. It is this form of interdependence that is best suited to a focused factory approach to health care delivery.

*Reciprocal* interdependence exists when two or more work processes or units mutually depend on each other in an interactive fashion in order for each to accomplish its task. Most processes involved in the delivery of health care services are of a reciprocally interdependent nature. For example, physicians are dependent on ancillary support services such as laboratory and radiology for results in order to treat the patient, and the ancillary support services are dependent on physicians for accurate test information. Each work unit may modify its behavior as a result of the behavior and information received from the other. In similar fashion, patients with chronic illness are frequently cared for by interdisciplinary teams that rely heavily on each other in order to carry out their tasks. Reciprocal interdependence requires the highest degree of integration activity. Written rules, instructions, guidelines, protocols, and focused factory approaches by themselves are inadequate to the task. They must be complemented by mutual adjustment processes characterized by face-to-face communication and the ability to adapt quickly to changing events.

The key lesson in this typology is the need to match the integration strategy to the required level of interdependence. This requires developing a portfolio approach to clinical integration management; a simplified example is shown in Table 5.1. An organized delivery system can implement these various strategies on an individual site-by-site basis or systemwide. Experience suggests that

Table 5.1. Portfolio Approach to Clinical
Integration Based on Level of Interdependence.

| Form of Interdependence | Examples | Relevant Clinical Integration Strategies |
|---|---|---|
| Pooled | Disease prevention Health promotion for well patients | Primary care physicians as "assemblers" and overseers of the process |
| Sequential | Acute care, single episode of illness (such as total hip replacement) | Guidelines, protocols, pathways |
| Reciprocal | Chronic illness (such as diabetes, or asthma, or congestive heart failure) | Case management, disease management |

the extent to which these strategies are used systemwide depends on the homogeneity of patient and population needs and preferences for care (Bower, 1998), as well as the geographic concentration of sites and the system's ability to standardize work processes and measurement of outcomes. The greater the homogeneity of patient needs and preferences, the greater the geographic concentration of sites, and the greater the system's ability to standardize care processes and measurement, the greater is the ability to deploy the portfolio of clinical integration strategies across the entire system. This results in the potential to achieve economies of both scale and scope. As Conrad (1993) has noted, "The essence of a system is the ability to aggregate up individual level care coordination and clinical processes into a system level capacity to plan, deliver, monitor, and adjust the structures and strategies for coordinating the care of populations over time. The coordination of care for individual patients is a necessary but not sufficient condition to realizing system level clinical integration" (p. 492). Others have found that when an organization reaches 30 percent managed care penetration in the population under age sixty-five and 15 percent penetration in the

Medicare risk population, there are real benefits to moving to a systemwide clinical integration strategy (Fowler and Stokes, 1996).

Necessary conditions for achieving clinical integration, therefore, are to (1) understand how clinical integration is influenced by overall corporate and managerial-level decision making as well as the design of work processes (the embeddedness concept) and (2) be able to assess the degree and type of interdependence required to care for different types of patients and match integration strategies to these different demands. Although these are necessary conditions, they are not sufficient. Based on the experience of the study systems over the past four years and existing literature, we have identified some additional likely key success factors and examples of some better practices. We have organized these within a framework of strategic, structural, cultural, and technical dimensions.

## Key Success Factors and Some Better Practices

Four dimensions influence organized delivery systems' ability to achieve clinical integration (O'Brien and others, 1995; Shortell and others, 1996):

> *Strategic dimension*—emphasizes that clinical integration must focus on strategically important issues facing the system, not on peripheral activities. Clinical integration must be seen as a core strategic priority of the system.
>
> *Structural dimension*—refers to the overall organizational structure of the system to support clinical integration efforts. This includes the use of committees, councils, task forces, work groups, service line management, and related arrangements for implementing and diffusing clinical integration efforts throughout the system.
>
> *Cultural dimension*—refers to the underlying beliefs, values, norms, and behavior of the system, which either supports or inhibits clinical integration work.

Technical dimension—refers to the extent to which people have the necessary training and skills to achieve clinical integration objectives. It also includes the organization's information technology capabilities.

In order to achieve a high degree of clinical integration, systems must attend to all four dimensions simultaneously and attempt to align them with each other. Table 5.2 suggests what happens when one or another dimension is missing.

As Table 5.2 suggests, when the strategic dimension is missing, nothing really important gets done. Clinical integration efforts have relatively little impact because they are not focused on the strategic priorities of the system. When the structural component is missing, one observes pockets of clinical integration success but little

Table 5.2. Components Needed to Achieve
Clinical Integration Across the Continuum of Care.

| Strategic | Structural | Cultural | Technical | Result |
|-----------|------------|----------|-----------|--------|
| 0 | 1 | 1 | 1 | No significant impact on anything really important |
| 1 | 0 | 1 | 1 | Inability to capture the learning and spread it throughout the organization |
| 1 | 1 | 0 | 1 | Small, temporary effects; no lasting impact |
| 1 | 1 | 1 | 0 | Frustration and false starts |
| **1** | **1** | **1** | **1** | **Lasting systemwide impact** |

Note: 1 = present; 0 = absent.
Source: Shortell and others (1996).

organizationwide or systemwide impact. This is because the structures for diffusing the learning and best practices throughout the organization and system are missing. When the cultural component is absent, nothing lasts. Short-run success falls apart because the organization lacks an overall culture that supports clinical integration work. No one recognizes it or rewards it on a daily basis. Absence of the technical dimension results in frustration and false starts because people do not have the necessary training in continuous improvement techniques necessary to support clinical integration work. It is only when all four dimensions are worked on simultaneously and aligned with each other that sustainable progress occurs. This is both the reason that achieving clinical integration is so difficult and, at the same time, a potentially powerful source of sustainable advantage.

## Key Strategic Success Factors

A number of strategic factors can be identified as important for clinical integration to be successful.

### Central Focus

Clinical integration must be seen as central to achieving the system's mission and its financial success. It must be a core component of the system's business plan. All of the study systems explicitly noted clinical integration as one of their system's strategic priorities. This was evident in both interviews of top management team members and reviews of written planning documents. As one CEO commented, "We have concentrated up to now on functional integration. We now want to take what we have done with functional integration and move the focus to clinical integration." Another CEO noted that "clinical integration is our next frontier."

One of the problems in pursuing clinical integration as a core strategy is in getting the buy-in from physicians, individual hospitals, and, where they exist, a system's own health plan. Everyone is supportive of clinical integration in principle and in the abstract, but implementation steps on nearly everyone's toes. Each of the major components of a health system—physicians, hospitals, and health plans—may have a different idea of what clinical integration means and how to achieve it. To physicians, it means well-coordinated patient care, whether a service is provided by a system operating unit or an entity outside the system. A given physician typically will have little interest or concern whether someone else's patients receive coordinated care or whether care is coordinated throughout the entire system. The challenge is to *get* the individual physician to identify with the larger organization and the larger population of patients for whom the organization bears some responsibility. Having physicians joined together into more grouplike practice organizations that are linked to the larger system through various arrangements such as PHOs and MSOs is one way of creating this larger sense of identity. Evolving research suggests that physicians who have greater identification with an organized delivery system are more likely to implement care management practices consistent with the system's integration strategy and are also more satisfied (Waters and others, 2000; Burns and others, 2000).

Individual hospitals interpret clinical integration as applying to patients in that hospital's service area. As such, the hospital may resist attempts to develop systemwide clinical integration initiatives because it may mean that it may have to give up some of its services and curtail its ability to operate autonomously. To overcome this barrier, several of the study systems created financial incentives for hospital cooperation. For example, most systems centralized capital allocation and operating cash flow. If certain financial targets were met, then all operating units shared in the rewards. Some systems also drew on physician leaders to push for systemwide clinical integration initiatives. For example, at the Franciscan Health System in Tacoma, Washington, a part of Catholic HealthCare Initiatives, a systemwide oncology service line was implemented led by a leader of one of the system's oncology groups. They defined three service line levels based on patient acuity and grouped resources around the three respective hospitals in the system. The least severe patients were treated at the small local community hospital, the more severe at the intermediate-size hospital, and the most severe at the large teaching-oriented hospital. Standardized protocols, criteria for referral and follow-up, and monitoring and accountability were all implemented.

A health plan's major objective is to keep employers happy with a given combination of benefits, premiums, and enrollee experience with care. Health plans support clinical integration efforts to the extent that they result in more cost-effective delivery of care for their subscribers. Where the enrollment base is large (for example, several hundred thousand lives and above), health plans can play a leadership role in developing and encouraging implementation of guidelines, protocols, disease management, and related care management practices. But often the plan does not have a sufficient number of enrollees to influence the practice behavior of individual physicians. Based on current fieldwork, respondents suggested that a physician needed to have approximately one-third of patients coming from a single payer source before the physician would begin to pay attention to implementing payer guidelines, protocols, and related care management practices. Lacking such influence, many plans attempt to micromanage physician behavior by mandating prior authorization, utilization management, drug formularies, and related techniques that frequently disrupt the continuity of patient care. Denial of a specific test, procedure, referral, or drug may save short-run costs but result in greater overall costs per episode of illness through repeat visits. In brief, many health plans do not take a sufficiently long-run view of their enrollees' situation in such a way as to promote and encourage clinical integration to take place. Even without a large base of health plan enrollees to influence clinical integration, several of the study systems attempted to deal with the issue through extensive involvement of the health plan's management team in all aspects of system operations. As the CEO of Sentara Healthcare noted, "I cannot go to a meeting without health plan people, hospital operations people, and physician group practice people being there. The health plan participates in every way."

*Explicit Implementation Plans*

Evidence that clinical integration is in fact central to the system's strategy can be found in execution. There must be a specific business plan that establishes priorities, allocates resources, and fixes accountability with a specific person over a specific period of time. Six of the nine systems had developed such plans in areas that include cardiovascular care, cancer care, orthopedics, women's health, and behavioral medicine. Mercy Health Services, among the first to develop such plans in 1996, has now expanded these efforts to cardiology, orthopedics, obstetrics, and oncology. Each of these is organized as a "knowledge-based care management process" (see the case study at the end of this chapter). Among the key facilitating factors in Mercy's progress has been experience in CQI, the importance of having a common vision and shared culture, the development of interdisciplinary teams, growing capability in information systems, and expanding clinical leadership (Porter, Van Cleave, and Milobowski, 1996). Advocate Health Care has also made progress in its clinical integration efforts. Building on early success in the management of congestive heart failure, it is now initiating a similar program for management of breast cancer and starting a systemwide patient safety initiative. Like Mercy, it stresses the importance of having strong clinical leadership in place, experience with CQI, and information systems that facilitate internal benchmarking.

*Performance Appraisal and Reward System*

A third important strategic success factor (although it can also be considered a structural factor) is the need to provide people with feedback on how well they are doing with clinical integration activities and reward them for achieving clinical integration objectives. Traditional performance appraisal and reward systems based on individual achievement alone are insufficient for evaluating clinical integration work, which is inherently a team effort. Skills in working within and across teams become an important area for development. Also, basing a higher percentage of an individual's pay on achievement of team objectives as opposed to individual objectives becomes necessary. A few study systems such as Sentara, Fairview, and Sutter Health were beginning to provide financial incentives for selected top management members who achieve specific clinical integration objectives.

### Population-Based Health Planning

It is difficult to plan and implement a continuum of services for a given population of people without knowing something about the likely demand for those services. This is true whether one is paid on a capitated basis, although the consequences for failing to match service capacity to demand are more severe the greater the degree is of capitated payment. Population-based planning requires information on the system's catchment area in regard to target groups by age, gender, socioeconomic status, and geography and identified specific subgroups that may be at risk for diabetes, asthma, congestive heart failure, substance abuse, violence, and related conditions. An example of such an approach is illustrated by the following comments of a Sutter physician:

> Our basic philosophy—you need to identify the population at risk in the first place before reacting to an event. If that's done, potentially capitated payment can make the integration better. The problem with managed care now that it is driven by utilization review and utilization management, which tends to limit resources rather than provide appropriate ones. If you start with a pooled-capped dollar, identify patients through population groups, and are flexible on how you provide services . . . then the potential is excellent.
>
> In the model we piloted here . . . all Medicare risk enrollees are screened initially with a risk identification tool. We break it out into four levels. Level three of

those at risk predominately need social support. They need Meals on Wheels, caregiver support, respite, someone to mow their lawn. That's triage through a community based social services network [Miller, Lipton, and Duke, 1997].

## Key Structural Success Factors

When Robert C. Parker, M.D., talks about care coordination, it almost sounds like a relay race: a series of carefully timed interrelated events whose outcome depends on a clear understanding of the situation at hand, efficiency, and good communication: "You've got a patient in the hospital today; he's not feeling well and they're trying to discharge him into a subacute care facility or into home care, or maybe you're trying to create a follow-up for him to be seen in a doctor's office or rehab," explains Parker, CEO of the Carle Clinic Association in Urbana, Illinois. "The challenge: how do you pass the baton across the continuum in a way that's efficient—without dropping the baton?" (Darby, 1999, p. 2).

Addressing Parker's challenge requires redesigning both the overall organization structure of a delivery system and its individual work processes. Overall structure can be divided into macro and micro levels. At the macro level are the overall governance and management processes that link facilities across a continuum of care, such as hospitals, physician clinic sites, long-term care facilities, and home health agencies. At the micro level are various arrangements established to coordinate care across delivery sites typically identified in the literature under various forms of service line management (Charns and Tewksbury, 1993).

Separate from these structural arrangements are efforts to redesign work flow activities associated with providing patient care; these are often referred to as process reengineering (Champy and Hammer, 1993). The experience of the study systems and others is that both overall organizational restructuring and work process reengineering are needed to promote clinical integration. Structural changes in organizational relationships or service line creation without recognizing the work flow of activities is a waste of time and resources. But systems have also learned that redesigning work processes without changing the structure within which these processes occur frequently results in suboptimization and short-term gains at best.

A prime example of a large-scale structural reorganization designed to achieve greater service level integration is the Veterans Administration's creation of vertically integrated service networks (VISNs). Results based on a study of fourteen VISNs found that 76 percent of clinical services have been structurally integrated as either consolidated or combined units with a perceived clinical impact of 3.8 (1 equals low and 5 equals high) and an operational impact of 3.5 (VanDeusen Lukas and Simon, 1998).

Many of the study systems have implemented clinical service lines over the past five years, but Inova Health System in Fairfax, Virginia, has ten years of experience with a cardiac care service line designed to integrate inpatient and postdischarge care for over twelve hundred patients. It has experienced steadily decreasing lengths of stay and patient satisfaction levels in the high ninetieth percentile (Darby, 1999). As an example of the linkage between the overall design of the service line concept and its specific work processes, Inova has identified five key criteria for success:

- The importance of preparing patients for what to expect. Patients receive pathway instructions in advance describing in lay terms what will happen to them at every step of the way.

- Developing a documentation system that travels with the patient throughout the continuum of care.

- Using standing orders and protocols to ensure uniformity of care from the operating room to the intensive care unit to the telemetry unit.

- Rearranging staffing to facilitate better patient communication and follow-up care.

- Establishing a strong link with home care. Home care nurses help patients stay on the pathway.

In regard to redesigning work processes, certain rules or guidelines can be used in combining services, functions, and activities. These guidelines take into account the degree of interdependence or relatedness of the services, functions, or activities involved. Services, functions, and activities can be usefully combined if they are clinically related, sociodemographically linked, or organizationally related. The guideline of clinical relatedness means combining activities that involve similar treatment inputs, practices, and approaches. These are particularly relevant in the area of high-technology acute care services.

Sociodemographic relatedness refers to the grouping of patients by such characteristics as age, sex, ethnicity, or income. These may apply to organizing care around women, senior citizens, Hispanic Americans, African Americans, and so on. Organizing around these characteristics tends to be more prevalent when dealing with primary care, disease prevention, and health promotion issues.

Organizationally related criteria include organizational structure, skill mix of personnel, and various logistical issues. The goal here is to achieve managerial economies of scope such that structure, personnel, and logistical support services are used to their best advantage.

Sometimes one guideline predominates, as in the case of cardiovascular disease, where the clinical approach comes to the forefront. In other situations, combinations of approaches may be needed, as in the case of breast cancer screening programs for women of targeted age groups. In still other cases, the guidelines may be in conflict with each other, as in the case of those who believe educational programs involving AIDS patients should be part of an overall community health educational initiative versus those who believe the programs ought to be targeted for separate attention. The goal in all cases, however, should be to organize care such that patients and community members experience the most continuous care possible with the best achievable outcomes using the fewest resources. Inevitably there will be some trade-offs across patient groups and community members because achieving cost-effective care for the greatest number of people is the goal and challenge of mass customization.

One potentially promising new approach to dealing with these issues is to focus on microsystems of care, defined as the smallest replicable unit of an organization required to deliver a service to a customer (Quinn, 1992). In the context of clinical integration, microsystems can be thought of as care teams organized to meet the needs of the patient. Some are using the microsystem concept in developing an idealized design for a clinical office practice (Berwick and Kilo, 1999). Table 5.3 provides a summary of relevant contrasting features between a typical clinical practice site and the idealized design.

Figure 5.2 then provides a checklist developed by Scripps Health in San Diego, California which systems can use to evaluate specific design efforts.

Table 5.3. Characteristics of Traditional
Versus Ideal Clinical Practice Sites.

| Classical Office | The Office We Need |
| --- | --- |
| Patients are scheduled into a fixed pattern of available care. | The pattern of supply is continually shaped to match better and better predictions of actual demand. |
| Waiting and queues are used to adjust for mismatches between supply and demand. | Prediction, flexibility, and contingency plans are used to reduce waits and queues to zero. |
| Medical records and other documents are designed for compliance and by habit; the record is chronological. | Medical records are continually shaped for usability and reduced in complexity; the record is problem oriented. |
| The medical record "belongs" to the clinical system. | The medical record "belongs" to the patient. |

Table 5.3. Characteristics of Traditional
Versus Ideal Clinical Practice Sites, Cont'd.

| Classical Office | The Office We Need |
|---|---|
| Office flow is segmented and unpredictable, and consists of individual tasks. | Office flow is continuous, predictable, and managed in teams. |
| Clinical care is based on individual training and habit; historical patterns are the "default" patterns; clinicians seek to preserve autonomy. | Clinical care is standardized when wise, and based on continually revised understandings of scientific evidence; best-known practices are the "default" patterns; clinicians seek to ensure consistency. |
| Clinicians make decisions about what is best for patients. | Each individual patient makes decisions about what is best for him or her, with the clinician as coach. |
| Clinicians access scientific knowledge, primarily in journals. | Clinicians and patients access scientific knowledge through any means. |
| Clinicians use their brains. | Clinicians use their brains, assisted by useful decision support and information systems in real time. |
| Leadership and management in the office are implicit, informal, and charismatic. | Leadership and management in the office are explicit, formal when useful, charismatic, and participative. |
| Financial performance is viewed as a matter of volume or not understood. | Financial performance is viewed as an optimization problem and well understood by all. |
| Staff development ceases at hiring; job descriptions are fixed. | Staff are "hired for attitude" and continually trained for new and broader skills and cross-functionality. |

*Source:* Berwick and Kilo (1999).

Figure 5.2.  Checklist for Assessing Care Redesign Efforts.

| Does It Improve: | No | Yes | Impact (1–5)[a] |
|---|---|---|---|
| Service responsiveness | | | |
| Patient outcomes | | | |
| Work environment | | | |
| Cost efficiency | | | |
| The entire experience seamless for the patient | | | |
| Simplify and/or streamline the process | | | |
| Revenue | | | |
| Percentage of time available for direct patient care | | | |
| Continuity of care | | | |

| Does It Reduce: | No | Yes | Impact (1–5)[a] |
|---|---|---|---|
| Costs | | | |
| Standby and wait time | | | |
| Number of people the patient interacts with | | | |
| Job boundaries | | | |
| Scheduling time/tasks | | | |
| Coordination time/tasks | | | |
| Documentation time/tasks | | | |
| Fragmented patient units | | | |
| The time the patient is unavailable to the caregiver | | | |
| Number of steps in the process | | | |

| Does It Improve: | No | Yes | Impact (1–5)[a] |
|---|---|---|---|
| Eliminate unnecessary work | | | |
| Nondirect patient care activities | | | |
| Patient transport time | | | |
| Specimen transport time | | | |
| Supply transport time | | | |
| Variation in the process | | | |
| Process redundancies | | | |
| Number of handoffs | | | |
| Average length of stay | | | |
| Risk of patient readmission | | | |

Figure 5.2. Checklist for Assessing Care Redesign Efforts, Cont'd.

| Does It Improve: | No | Yes | Impact (1–5)[a] |
|---|---|---|---|
| The distances walked by key ancillary personnel | | | |
| Number of incumbents per job class | | | |

| Does It Increase: | No | Yes | Impact (1–5)[a] |
|---|---|---|---|
| The skills, knowledge, and abilities of caregivers | | | |
| Use of employee skills and training | | | |
| Broadens job definitions | | | |
| Patient satisfaction | | | |
| Physician satisfaction | | | |
| Employee satisfaction | | | |
| Percentage of care at or near bedside | | | |
| Caregivers' control over care provided | | | |

| Does It Provide: | No | Yes | Impact (1–5)[a] |
|---|---|---|---|
| Easily quantifiable results | | | |
| A changed organization structure | | | |
| Focused patient populations | | | |
| The right thing is done right the first time by the right person | | | |
| Consolidate work functions | | | |
| A redesigned process | | | |
| An integrated team whose mission and loyalty are to the patient | | | |
| Compliance to daily and discharge clinical outcomes | | | |
| For services to be provided closer to the patient | | | |

[a]1 = low; 5 = significant.

*Source:* Scripps Health, San Diego, Calif., 1999.

In considering the microsystem and related concepts, it is important to realize that meeting the needs of many patients, particularly those with chronic illness, requires that microsystems be linked together as part of overall care systems. Further, to improve population health requires the linkage of care systems with other community organizations that share a common vision and purpose.

## Key Cultural Success Factors

To accomplish clinical integration requires a culture that is end results oriented, learning oriented, and change oriented. Emerging research suggests that group practices affiliated with organized delivery systems in which the group has a culture that is achievement and end results oriented demonstrate greater implementation of care management practices and accountability (Shortell, Zazzali, Burns, and others, 2000). But most study systems found it difficult to encourage these attributes consistently due to the "multicultural" nature of the various groups and units making up an organized delivery system. Although individual hospitals, physician groups, and health plans shared some common values, they also had their own distinct cultures, which often influenced whether, how, and at what speed desired changes would or could occur. Further, cultural differences often existed within these units. As a result, it was difficult for the study systems to build momentum toward achieving widespread clinical integration, particularly lacking payment or market incentives to do so. Nonetheless, three factors identified in our earlier work continue to play an important role in facilitating clinical integration: a strong commitment to CQI/TQM, training of multiskilled workers, and development of clinical leadership.

### CQI/TQM Commitment

CQI/TQM approaches are ideally suited for the types of complex reciprocal work processes associated with coordinating patient care across providers and sites over time. CQI/TQM provides a skill set, a common language, and, perhaps most important, a philosophical and conceptual framework for achieving clinical integration. Most of the study systems had been implementing CQI/TQM since the early 1990s and over the past four years have engaged in considerable experimentation in their approaches. These have been characterized by more direct application to clinical conditions and processes and by quicker, more targeted interventions. CQI/TQM processes have been used to implement new evidence-based medical findings in regard to clinical guidelines, protocols, pathways, care management, and disease management approaches. Most systems are also using systems' thinking principles, working backward from the desired end state to systematically examining the causal chain that influences the desired end state (Churchman, 1974; Ackoff, 1979). Most are also using rapid cycle process improvement principles based on the plan, do, study, and act (PDSA) approach (Langley and others, 1996).

Among the most salient advantages of CQI/TQM noted by the study systems was that of providing a common language for improvement. Every study system indicated that exposing people to CQI/TQM training philosophies and practices was essential for doing clinical integration work. It provided a means through which people could communicate with each other, gather and analyze data on what services might best be combined, decide on the most efficient series of steps for providing a service, and develop process and outcome measures for assessing performance. For example, over the past four years alone, Henry Ford Health System has trained over one thousand physicians and employees in TQM practices and principles. This has served as a foundation for its clinical process improvement work in cervical cancer screening, lab testing, joint replacement, obstetrics, asthma care, and other areas. As one Ford employee noted, "Today it's hard to imagine significant progress in improving clinical services without this cultural shift supported by total quality management" (Henry Ford Health System, 1993).

Fairview's clinical integration work has been based in large part on five CQI core beliefs: (1) focus on individual leadership, (2) focus on customers, (3) focus on process, (4) focus on people, and (5) focus on measurement. These have been translated into examples for every employee, and each employee's performance is measured by how effectively he or she has demonstrated the behavior in action on a seven-point scale, from ineffective to effective. Examples of ineffective performance include "fails to understand how actions and decisions affect others' work or business as a whole," "focuses only on traditional areas of responsibility," "operates independently from the team," and "resists the input and assistance from others." Examples of positive behavior include "takes a systematic approach to resolving problems and issues," "recognizes that customer needs and expectations extend beyond department boundaries," "seeks to remove processes not required to meet customer expectations," and "functions as an integral team member." The case studies at the end of this chapter provide further examples of the role played by CQI/TQM in achieving meaningful levels of clinical integration.

### New Training for New Workers

Clinical integration depends on developing multiskilled workers who take a holistic view of the patient and the continuum of care required to maintain, enhance, or restore the patient's health. Although this could just as readily be considered a technical success factor, the key here is the cultural value of wholeness, integration, and empowerment. Multiskilled professionals who can operate in teams and keep a clear focus on customer requirements contribute to developing the holographic organization in which the whole is embedded in each part. Several systems were making major efforts in cross-training as part of their CQI/TQM and clinical reengineering work.

An important feature of multiskilled training is adopting a philosophy of continuous learning. The organizations furthest along in cross-training and multiskilled training used every opportunity that arose in the course of doing daily work as an opportunity for learning. Reports on lessons learned were built into every team meeting, and great reliance was placed on developing self-teaching modules.

Performance appraisal criteria were developed in which an individual did not receive credit for learning a new skill until he or she had taught it or shared it with someone else. Incentives for participating in advanced CQI/TQM training were created whereby individuals received credit only if all team or unit members attended. These represent examples of building a learning organization (Senge, 1990; Huber and Glick, 1993) and are seen as essential to clinical integration. Following is an example of how such training and learning works at the micro level:

> Developing guidelines is a complex process. It involves training and forms, revision and reconfiguration of scheduling and information systems—an enormous number of activities. In our system, this process involves some 5,000 front line and support staff. Hundreds of daily encounters occur in 50 locations, each with its own ways of scheduling, of handling what patient information is dispensed, how it's dispensed, how nurses and doctors interact, who does what.
>
> For example, suppose you want to implement the bladder infection protocol. You go to the physician's office and you sit down with the nurse and the doctor who [is] in a larger practice with five doctors and a couple of nurses and the receptionist—and you ask, "What's your current process for managing a bladder infection?"
>
> There is a little pause, and the head nurse looks at you and says, "For which doctor?"
>
> And then you say "Well, let's pick Dr. Jones." And she says, "Well, Dr. Jones is fairly new here, and he set up a system with those little three by five cards. We've got them in a box by the phone. We just look up bladder infection, and here's what it says: 'Come in, give us a urinalysis and culture. See the doctor."
>
> So how do you usually put this guideline to work in a pre-existing system like this one? You use what you've got.

You embed the guideline on that three by five card. If they've got some other kind of system—computer scheduling system reminders—you incorporate it there. That's the key to making it happen. That's what "do" is all about.

That same process has to happen for literally every physician throughout the system of 50 different practices. A lot of people's time is taken up in these difficult labor intensive implementation activities. That's where we have to count on the commitment and motivation of the medical groups and the organizations. . . .

Why do physicians and nurses take this on, and what keeps them going? It's not money, because we don't add a lot of money to the system for this. I think what keeps people doing this is that we start to generate an interesting learning engine. Physicians and nurses are trained scientifically, and many of them harbor a lot of curiosity. Does what they do in practice work or doesn't it?

This process is giving them a mechanism to start answering some questions that they wondered about for 20 years of practice. I wouldn't minimize the importance of this kind of motivation. It's what's going to sustain us over the long haul [Reinertsen, J. "Living Guidelines." *Healthcare Forum Journal*, Nov.–Dec. 1994, pp. 58–59. Reprinted by permission of Jossey-Bass Inc., a subsidiary of John Wiley & Sons, Inc.].

*Clinical Leadership Development*

Based on emerging knowledge regarding the effective functioning of microsystems, eight characteristics have been identified to promote clinical integration work (Povar and Shortell, 1999):

1. Developing a shared vision for team members so that they know how the vision is embedded in their own jobs on a daily basis

2. Understanding and acting on patient and population needs for the broad range of care that they may require

3. Having technical competence across the range of health and medical care and needs, including psychosocial aspects of care

4. Ensuring that all team members and the team as a whole understand the nature of its work processes, such as the demands for interdependence

5. Understanding and respect for each other's roles

6. Managing conflict effectively

7. Managing change effectively

8. Having available information to evaluate performance and take correct or improvement action.

It is important to note that seven of these eight (the exception being item three) are skills and attitudes that most physicians, nurses, and many other health professionals are not exposed to during their education and training. Therefore, they must be learned on the job. Over the past four years, study systems have made increasing investment in formally organized programs to develop such clinical leadership. Although most of these have been aimed at physicians, many have taken a team approach to include nurses and nonclinical managers as well. The goal is to develop clinical leaders who understand patient care from a population-based perspective, understand patients from a holistic perspective, understand care delivery from a continuum of care perspective, understand and are able to operate in teams and promote teamwork throughout the organization, know how to manage change and conflict, can link one microsystem to another, and understand how to use information systems for process improvement as well as for producing outcome measures for external accountability purposes. Almost all systems were incorporating content in most of the above areas into their leadership development programs.

### Key Technical Success Factors

Study systems have learned that you cannot improve that which you do not understand. Understanding requires data or observations that can be turned into information for generating knowledge. Thus, information systems are one of the most important technical success factors for clinical integration. The other is the technical and conceptual set of skills associated with reengineering.

*Information Systems*

For purposes of promoting clinical integration, the key aspects of information systems are their ability to link data from one encounter to another, from one provider to another, and from one site to another over time. Some of the data that the multiple caregivers need is generic and can be standardized, such as demographic information, basic health status, and drug allergies. But some of it will be specific to a condition or problem. The implication is that the design of information systems must be closely tied to an understanding of clinical medicine and clinical decision making. Although this point seems self-evident, the experience of the study systems is that it is difficult to implement in practice.

Although it is common to compare the health care sector with the banking and airlines industry in the use of electronic information to improve client service, the comparison is mostly unfair. It fails to recognize that most of the "encounter knowledge" in banking and airline transactions is easily codified, understandable, and routinized information, such as dates, times, and dollar amounts. In contrast, much of the information in clinical patient-physician interactions is tacit or uncodified knowledge, which is often difficult to communicate in a way that will be consistently meaningful to others (Teece, 1981, 1998). Such knowledge is more susceptible to errors of interpretation and therefore is more conducive to face-to-face communication. The challenge of promoting clinical integration through the use of more sophisticated information systems lies in striking a balance between the incorporation of medical knowledge that can be codified into electronic transfer of information that has meaning for other caregivers and knowledge that cannot be easily expressed or communicated electronically. This is aside from issues related to capital investment and information technology, patient confidentiality issues, and perceived resistance of professionals to using computerized patient records in their offices.

With these issues in mind, most study systems have devoted considerable capital, time, and energy to improving their information systems over the past four years. Most have, wisely, first attempted to answer questions related to what information is needed by whom, for what purpose, and at what point in time. They have also assessed the amount, type, and format of current data collected with the goal of streamlining before automating. A major focus has been on developing and implementing computerized patient records in physician offices.

Efforts at creating a longitudinal electronic record are not limited to the United States. One of the more interesting initiatives is associated with the Coordinated Care Trials in Australia (Ross, Mackey, and Herrick, 1998). Nine trials have been formed with the purpose of coordinating care for people with multiple needs based on the development of explicit care plans and the pooling of resources across different agencies. Critical to the success of this effort is the development of a longitudinal record containing four levels of information:

- Client-level data that link the client to the care plan, the care coordinator, and related caregivers

- Trial management data that monitor utilization, costs, and movement between services

- Evaluation data that track demographic details, service use, functional health status scores, costs, and morbidity

- Local implementation data related to the way the trial has been established, the impact on participating clients, and changes as a result of the care coordination interventions

*Reengineering*

Although reengineering may be viewed by some as a fad and by others as a euphemism for "slash and burn" cost cutting that leaves people without jobs, it continues to be an important success factor for most of the study systems in achieving clinical integration. An analogy can be made between growing a healthy organization and growing a healthy tree or beautiful garden. Occasionally trees and gardens need to be pruned and cut back to allow space for water, light, and air. So it is that healthy organizations also need to prune and rearrange to meet changing customer and stakeholder demands.

Reengineering in a sense goes beyond CQI/TQM by recognizing that some processes, programs, and services may require more than continuous improvement of existing behavior or reductions in variation; they may instead require total elimination and redesign. The difference is largely a matter of degree, but it is important nevertheless because reengineering often runs into more vocal political opposition within the organization. The scope of change is often much more pervasive in reengineering relative to CQI/TQM—in part, because CQI/TQM has not yet totally permeated most study systems' work or activities.

In our earlier work, we documented the efforts of several study systems in reengineering. For example, Sentara eliminated its department of physical therapy, reassigning its functions to nurses and other therapists. It also redesigned pharmacy in such a way that it eliminated the inpatient pharmacy department and redeployed the people who staffed it as pharmaceutical service managers who use their skills to help manage patients across the care continuum. These efforts continue.

As an example from outside the study systems, HealthSystem Minnesota's experience in reengineering cancer care is instructive (Appleby, 1997). Dr. David Abelson described the situation in the beginning as "a mess." "The rules, if any, are in the staff's heads." Using business reengineering techniques, Abelson and Dr. Linda Peitzman developed a formal clinical integration effort called Care

2000 composed of eight full-time and seventy part-time staff and drawing on an outside consultant with process engineering experience at the National Aeronautics and Space Administration and the U.S. Air Force. The cancer program encompassed a hospital-based unit, a home health agency with a hospice, two outpatient IV/chemotherapy sites, a six-physician outpatient clinic, one solo medical practice, and bone marrow transplant, pastoral care, and music therapy programs. In addition, there were forty-seven different computer systems and fifty different medical records with information. The goal was to develop a common health care information technology infrastructure that included the following components:

- Clinical data repository to give doctors customized displays of patient information over the Internet

- Electronic routing of patient data to everyone involved in the registration process

- A program that will allow doctors to order tests and drugs in line with electronic alerts about adverse drug reactions

- A computer form for patient education that will have multimedia presentations linked to the intranet

The system has invested $19 million in the effort. Prior to making these changes, patients were typically asked for the same information by seven different doctors and staff.

HealthSystem Minnesota's reengineering experience is based on a specific condition: cancer care. However, some systems are also making efforts to reengineer basic core processes of patient treatment such as the office visit. Modern electronic techniques in the form of the Internet make it increasingly possible to replace the traditional office visit as the major way of meeting health care needs. This will save time for both providers and patients and allow providers to spend more time with patients who require face-to-face interaction. Here is a fictional example of such an encounter:

*The patient's name is Marsha; a 78 year old female with congestive heart failure, hypertension, arthritis, seasonal affective disorder [SAD], widowed, and residing in an assisted living facility.*

At 9:45 A.M., Dr. Sosa and Marsha had their quarterly three month's visit for the purpose of monitoring her clinical status and provide ongoing health consultation. Before starting the TWIV-C visit [two-way interactive videoconferencing], scheduled for 30 minutes, Dr. Sosa reviewed the patient-capped, doctor-shared electronic medical record to review body weight, blood pressure, arthritis impact measurement (AIM scores), and mental health scores (all time-trended data on control charts showing the values for Marsha vis-à-vis age-sex relevant cohorts). Dr. Sosa also reviewed the list of questions and bothersome symptoms that Marsha had added to her list (to mention to Dr. Sosa over the past several weeks). Marsha, sitting in her living room and using TWIV-C, told Dr. Sosa that she was feeling "great" all things considered, and that she felt like she was doing a good job of controlling her weight and blood pressure and managing her arthritis but with winter coming she was concerned about dipping into depression. Dr. Sosa and Marsha discussed this concern and together they built an action plan that would increase the odds of preventing SAD. Their visit concluded at 10:10 with five minutes to spare. Marsha rated her visit with Dr. Sosa a nine on a zero to ten scale; her only concern was, will my anti-SAD plan work? [Scherger and Nelson, 1999].

There appear to be three keys to successful reengineering efforts. The first is for the organization to have some experience with CQI/TQM. No health care organization has successfully achieved reengineering without it. Second, it is important to select core processes for reengineering work in order to achieve demonstrable improvement in clinical integration and any possible attendant cost reductions. In other fields, it is estimated that reengineering a minor process or single activity has only a 1 percent effect on the bottom line; reengineering a core process or several interdependent processes can realize a 3 to 5 percent payoff; reengineering the entire organization might have as much as a 17 percent effect (Hall, Rosenthal, and Wade, 1993). Third is the need for strong information system technologies that include an open architecture, the ability to network, and database design (Kralovec, 1994). Reengineering draws on a health care organization's information strengths. Organizations that report some success in their reengineering efforts appear to be those with a more advanced ability to manage information such as the Henry Ford and Intermountain health systems (Griffith, Sahney, and Mohr, 1995).

## Future Issues: Chronic Illness

The major challenge for organized delivery systems in achieving greater levels of clinical integration for patients with chronic illness is to organize a coordinated array of services that meet patient and family member needs, as the following comments reflect:

> You're not going to be able to improve your care of an older, sicker population just because you manage adverse risk selection or do a better job as an insurance company. What you've got to be able to do is to deliver care more effectively [Wong, 1998, p. 12].

> In most respects, the waiting room at the health center that Marty Lynch directs is typical of any other community clinic: walls posted with notices announcing health education classes and receptionists busy on telephones.
>
> But there is one striking difference: all of the patients in the room are older people—some readily mobile, some

using walkers or canes, some very frail and accompanied by adult children.

At the over 60 Health Center in Berkeley, patients are waiting to see physicians, podiatrists, dentists, psychologists, and social workers at what amounts to the medical equivalent of one stop shopping.

Lynch, the clinic's executive director, sees his facility as a harbinger of things to come as the California health care profession recreates itself to care for the nation's largest population of elderly people. . . .

[Meanwhile, at the UCLA Medical Center in Los Angeles,] most of [Dr. David] Reuben's patients are 75 to 95 years old. As he states, "They are what today's healthy 65 year olds will look like in 20 years: frail, many with hip fractures, dementia, problems with mobility, balance, and urinary incontinence," he said. "These are the kinds of things every doctor will have to manage" [Perkins, 1999].

The experiences of the study systems and others around the country suggest that this will require the use of interdisciplinary teams trained in geriatric medicine, use of innovative case management programs, and the support of strong information systems. It is not a challenge likely to be met by focused factories, isolated microsystems, or carved-out disease management programs. As others have noted, "The basic idea is that [carve-outs] are good for illnesses that are rare, complicated, easily defined, and very costly, and that are somewhat isolated—that is, they don't entail multi-system illnesses. . . . Conversely for common multi-system illnesses that are not terribly complicated, not rare, and tend to be associated with many problems simultaneously, carve outs don't make a lot of sense" (Blumenthal, quoted in "Single Specialty Carve-outs: A Threat to Integrated Care," *Medical Network Strategy Report*, 1999). Others note: "If you're doing managed care correctly, you should be integrating specialties and carve out is *dis-integrating* care. . . . This is often a negotiating ploy for specialists rather than an effort to collaboratively improve care quality and care costs" (McDermott, quoted in "Single Specialty Carve-outs: A Threat to Integrated Care," *Medical Network Strategy Report*, 1999).

Study systems and others around the country are making only incremental progress in meeting the needs of people with chronic illness. In 1995, Fairview Health System formally affiliated with the Ebenezer Society, a comprehensive long-term care organization, in order to pursue its objectives of better managing care for the chronically ill. Using a self-assessment for systems integration (SASI) tool developed by the National Chronic Care Consortium, the Fairview-Ebenezer partnership has resulted in some perceived improvements in infrastructure, communication systems, care management, coordination, and client involvement. Nonetheless, on a scale from 0 (low) to 4 (high), most of these scores are in the 2.0 to the 2.5 range. As noted by Richard Norling, Fairview CEO, in 1997: "When one examines the continuum of services required of patients with chronic illnesses, most of these programs will be delivered in non-acute care settings. An overly-Hospital-Centric viewpoint will clearly be a hindrance to a system committed to developing integrated chronic-care services" ("Case Study . . . ," 1997, p. 2).

Sisters of Providence Health System has also made considerable efforts to integrate care for the chronically ill, particularly in the Portland, Oregon, region. In this region, it has a single management structure and a single strategic plan along with bottom-line financial responsibility for hospitals, long-term care, hospice care, PACE (Program of All-inclusive Care of the Elderly), and an assisted living facility.

An example outside the study system is Group Health Cooperative of Puget Sound (Coberly, 1998). In 1997, in collaboration with the Center for Health Studies MacColl Institute for Health Care Innovation, Group Health launched an initiative to develop a number of chronic care clinics, beginning with diabetes. Common elements included a half-day session with similar patients and a grouping of providers, services, and equipment; standardized clinical and health assessments; implementation of guidelines; one-on-one visits with health teams as needed; patient education and support groups; and systematic follow-up. The initiative has faced many barriers, particularly as the Group Health Cooperative has faced financial problems and has had to cut back staff. Although it has yet to document the cost benefit of moving to this approach, it is seeing an increase in such intermediate measures as the number of diabetics whose feet are examined. It has also served as a testing ground to refine the approach to treating chronic illness resulting in the development of a chronic care management model (Wagner and others, 1999). The model has six key components (see Figure 5.4):

- Identifying community resources to support chronic care management and coordinating planning with the community

- Explicit incorporation of chronic care goals into the health system's annual business plan based on population-based planning, provider incentives, and effective performance improvement principles

- Programs emphasizing patient self-management and support resources for patient self-management

- Strong decision support systems including evidence-based guidelines and protocols and merging the expertise and knowledge of generalists and specialists

- Designing the delivery system to work together with the patient in anticipating problems

- Development of a clinical information system that includes a registry of patients with chronic conditions, reminder systems for patients and the care team, and the provision of regular feedback.

Figure 5.4. Chronic Care Management Model,
Group Health Cooperative of Puget Sound.

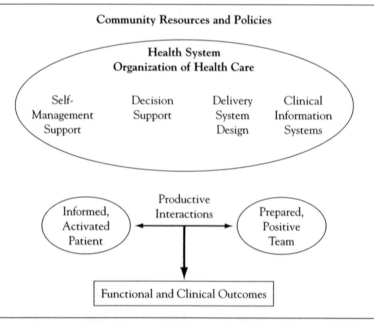

*Source:* Reprinted with permission from Wagner. E., and others. "A Survey of
Leading Chronic Disease Management Programs: Are They Consistent with the
Literature?" *Managed Care Quarterly,* 1999, 7(3), 56–66. Seattle, Wash.: MacColl
Center for Innovation and Health Promotion, 1999.

This model is currently being used in a national evaluation program designed to improve chronic illness for patients with congestive heart failure, diabetes, depression, and care for the frail elderly
(Robert Wood Johnson Foundation, 2000).

The above experiences are also consistent with the PACE (Program of All-Inclusive Care of the Elderly) and SHMO-2 (Social
Health Maintenance Organization) programs (Boult and Pacala,
1999). These initiatives attempt to integrate acute and long-term
care and have received support from the Health Care Financing
Administration. The evidence that these programs are either cost-
effective or cost-beneficial, however, is still largely lacking (Kane

and others, 1997; Harrington, Lynch, and Newcomer, 1993; Harrington and Newcomer, 1991; Manton and others, 1993).

Overall, clinical integration for the management of people with chronic illness is still largely a promise in search of performance. On the one hand, it is difficult to argue with Wilensky (1997) who notes, "It is hard to imagine a system that would be better designed to deliver appropriate high quality care than one that incorporates the full continuum of care. The power of an integrated patient care (IPC) system to achieve proper trade-offs and make the best use of the whole care continuum makes the notions of carve outs, sub-capitated systems, and horizontal integration pale by comparison." That is the promise. Zelman (1996) best summarizes the performance to date: "But the existence of capability and potential for positive change are no guarantee that the potential will be achieved. Today, that potential, especially with regard to clinical integration and quality of care remains largely untapped. And there is no certainty that it will be fully tapped" (p. 305). In the words of one of our study system's CEOs, "It is primarily still a price game and not a patient care integration game."

### Henry Ford Health System: Partnership in Pregnancy and Parenting

Henry Ford Health System (HFHS) is engaged in a number of initiatives designed to achieve greater clinical integration of care for its patients across the continuum of care. One of these is the Partnership in Pregnancy and Parenting Program (PIPP), which provides a continuum of education and support for new mothers from the earliest months of pregnancy through the baby's first year. Rather than focus on the acute (inpatient) birth episode as is traditional, PIPP offers intense education and home health visits in combination with a shortened hospital stay. Even though it may have started as a program, today PIPP is simply the highest standard of care that HFHS leaders hope will serve as a model for other episodes of care and quality improvement initiatives.

PIPP grew out of dissatisfaction with an earlier effort that emphasized a voluntary short-stay maternity program. This program was plagued by inconsistent care and variances in implementation. The philosophy behind the new program was captured in the following statement:

> An opportunity exists for the Henry Ford Medical Group to be proactive and define a short-stay program that could become the standard for obstetrical care before it becomes defined for us by third-party payors. The program would reduce the standard stay to one day for vaginal deliveries and would incorporate a carefully planned system of education and support so that our patients could be discharged with specific knowledge and skill base as well as qualified home support. It is the belief of the team that such a program would result in knowledgeable, confident patients who would be more satisfied with their obstetrical experience.

### The Program

At the outset, team members identified three stages of care—prenatal, inpatient, and home care—and began to develop clinical pathways for each stage.

*Prenatal assessment.* At twenty-eight to thirty-two weeks, PIPP participants meet with an ob/gyn nurse specialist who assesses the patient's educational soundness, reviews the material presented in handouts, and evaluates her physical and social status. The assessment includes a physical exam and a variety of questions to determine if the patient is mentally prepared for childbirth and can demonstrate a sufficient knowledge base for the stage of pregnancy. The assessment tool includes a checklist of possible indicators for a home health referral. These include suspicion of substance or spousal abuse, expectant mothers below age eighteen years, high-risk pregnancy, and lack of knowledge related to infant care or pregnancy. A nurse who discovers or suspects any problems recommends a predelivery home visit to help the family prepare to care for the new baby. If adequate preparations cannot be made in the patient's home, the nurse can advise against early discharge. [Adapted from: "Partnership in Pregnancy and Parenting," *Innovations in Organized Systems of Care.*]

*Inpatient care.* Inpatient clinical pathways define the process for labor and delivery as well as the twenty-four hours postpartum (three days for cesarean section) for both the mother and baby. The PIPP team suggested two changes in existing practices for inpatient care. First, circumcisions are to be done earlier; they had previously been performed one hour before discharge. Second, the team developed protocols to ensure that newborn screening would occur a second time during a home health care visit if it had occurred in the hospital before the baby was twenty-four hours old. For example bilirubin screening does not always yield accurate results in the first twenty-four hours, so a second screening is often warranted.

*Home health care.* The clinical pathways for home health care visits specify the timing and content of each visit. The first is to occur within twenty-four hours of discharge and the second two to three days later. The timing of these visits is based on what pediatricians feel is the best time to detect specific problems in the newborn. During the visits, the home health nurse conducts physical examinations of both mother and baby. The nurse determines if the uterus is firm and how much bleeding is occurring, and also takes a blood sample and performs a test for phenylketonuria (pku). Test results are provided the same day and discussed with the physician. The nurse and patient discuss breast-feeding and review other issues, and the mother receives her final educational handout ("Learning to Parent"). All home health nurses have extensive experience and are especially credentialed in the care of mothers and babies.

## Implementation

After piloting PIPP at the Fairlane Center (one of Henry Ford's health centers) for a six-month period, team members made several changes before the program was implemented across the system.

First, the pediatric staff members were given the educational materials and included in provider focus groups for ongoing program evaluation. Next, some restructuring was done on the prenatal education classes, which are taught by contracted nurses and nurse midwives. These nurse contractors provided their thoughts on the substance of the educational materials, and their classes were restructured so that all materials were presented in the PIPP format. Finally, a full-time project coordinator was assigned to implement the project at other sites. After these changes, PIPP was rolled out at other sites, starting with the HFHS main campus and moving to the satellite clinics, Henry Ford hospitals, and, finally, contracted hospitals.

At each site, implementation began with extensive orientation sessions. The project coordinator met staff at each clinical site to answer questions, address concerns, and facilitate implementation. This person also brought an inpatient PIPP-trained nurse as well as a PIPP-trained home health nurse. Nurses and physicians, including ob/gyns, pediatricians, and family practitioners, were encouraged to accompany a home health nurse on a home visit.

Much of the implementation process was focused on getting professionals to begin thinking about maternity care in a process-oriented fashion. Although process compliance was emphasized, sites were allowed some flexibility in assigning responsibility for managing the PIPP process. A concurrent case management system was employed to help with the transition to process-oriented care. Case management enables the care of every patient to be monitored and documented as she moves through each clinical pathway: outpatient, inpatient, and home care. Variation from pathways is documented and fed back to each department, which has allowed the PIPP project team to make improvements to the process and given providers the information they needed to modify their practices.

### Barriers to Implementation

The PIPP project team encountered several obstacles during implementation. As expected, physicians and nurses expressed concern about early discharge. They were particularly concerned that there might not be adequate time to educate the mother and that the infant assessments might not take place as they should. During orientation and follow-up meetings, the project team emphasized that PIPP actually exceeded services traditionally offered, especially in the areas of patient education, one-on-one home health visits, and the benefits of recovering and learning in a more comfortable environment. Some clinicians went on PIPP home health visits and were reassured that mothers' and babies' needs were being met. These clinicians, especially the family physicians, were quickly convinced that PIPP works.

The majority of HFHS physicians are salaried employees; thus, there was more immediate buy-in on their part because they were comfortable following quality improvement processes to achieve cost-effectiveness goals. As expected, contract physicians were most resistant to the program. This created an unexpected problem in the hospital setting. In the early days of implementation, it was common for one hospital roommate to be getting the PIPP home health care visits and the other not. The roommate who was not under PIPP care would often question why she was not receiving these services. Such situations were inconsistent with the system's vision to create "brand-name" care.

The fact that PIPP was a "local initiative," as opposed to a leadership directive, was another obstacle to implementation. Although PIPP had a local physician champion, the program had no official nod of approval from physician leadership, so its implementation and acceptance were relatively uneven at first. When Dr. Thomas Royer came to HFHS as chief medical officer in 1994, he became the corporate sponsor of PIPP and pushed for systemwide implementation. Not long after that, PIPP was implemented across all HFHS sites.

Aside from the underlying pressure to provide high-quality, low-cost care, purchasers were not involved in establishing PIPP. It was primarily an internal initiative driven by a variety of factors, particularly the desire to reduce variation and increase quality of care. PIPP was also driven by the preferences of female patients who desired a more holistic birth experience, with less emphasis on inpatient hospitalization.

## Outcomes to Date

PIPP has been in place since 1996 and has shown impressive results. Perhaps most significant is the extent to which PIPP has been accepted by providers and patients. The majority of physicians are comfortable with the program, and many contract physicians have requested the PIPP educational materials and orientation. Moreover, other health care systems have expressed an interest in PIPP; some have even offered to purchase the PIPP materials.

Surveys and anecdotal experience reveal that patients value PIPP. "Repeat customers" often specifically request PIPP by name. They view the additional educational materials and one-on-one nurse interaction in the home as added benefits. . . . PIPP patients get much more intense care than they would ever get in the hospital. She also points out that mistakes are much more likely to occur in the hospital setting than at home, where one nurse is concentrating on one patient. Royer agrees, noting that the hospital, which has increasingly become oriented to tertiary care, "is not a place for the well or walking wounded."

According to Dr. Royer, PIPP has achieved the following results:

- Consistency of maternal and child health care has been achieved with defined expectations for physicians, support staff, and patients.

- PIPP has laid the groundwork and provided a model for clinical process improvement in other areas of patient care.

- PIPP has saved money. Despite the fact that HFHS has experienced increased outpatient and home health costs, the program saves about eighty to one hundred dollars per delivery on approximately five thousand births in the HFHS each year. As the program becomes more efficient and as other payers agree to pay for home health benefits provided under PIPP, savings are expected to increase.

- PIPP has developed a standard of care that can be taught to future physicians. Its emphasis on process consistency is particularly useful in a teaching hospital.

- PIPP has built morale and given local clinicians recognition from system leadership and the media.

In the beginning, PIPP project team members decided they would measure improvements based on four outcomes:

- Increased patient satisfaction with the care process

- Increased patient preparedness for pregnancy, childbirth, and parenting

- Stable clinical quality indicators (such as no increase in maternal or infant readmissions)

- Decreased length of hospital stay

PIPP has performed well on each of these key performance indicators. Patient satisfaction is higher since PIPP has been implemented. Pilot participants indicated (through a written survey administered at key points in the pregnancy) that they had read the materials, that materials were understandable and useful, and that they felt well prepared and knowledgeable.

To determine if shorter hospital stays are safe, HFHS conducted a study to examine rates of hospital readmission in conjunction with birth. They studied 1,775 women who have had short-stay deliveries since the implementation of PIPP and determined that readmission rates since PIPP's implementation were not significant. Of these, seventy-five infants remained in the hospital at the time of the mother's discharge, thirty-one infants were readmitted by day 14, and eight mothers were readmitted by day 14. Most readmissions occur days

4 and 5 and beyond, and not on days 2 or 3, which might indicate a problem with early discharges.

## Lessons Learned

Henry Ford's experience with PIPP highlights a number of lessons specific to the program itself as well as some more general to clinical integration efforts overall.

- Women need education and support for the changes of pregnancy and the immediate postpartum period; however, the stress and fatigue of childbirth make the hospital stay the least effective time to teach. Health systems should standardize educational materials and develop a distribution schedule that corresponds to the expectant mother's needs, because it is during this prepartum period that women will be able to absorb the most information and make many of the necessary preparations for birth. For the postpartum period, the home setting is a better learning environment, and it affords more time and hands-on instruction from the caregiver for the new mother to learn how to care for a newborn.

- To sustain momentum in a quality improvement effort, team members much be clear about the program's aim and have a deep personal commitment. In addition to a physician champion, these types of initiatives should include a directive from the system's top leadership and should be pursued in the context of a broader quality improvement effort.

- The pediatric staff should be involved early in the development of maternal and child health tools. They have valuable expertise, and their buy-in is important to the program's success.

- Systems should assess their needs and capacity before embarking on any major quality or process improvement initiative. It is difficult to implement systemwide process change without corresponding changes to the infrastructure. For instance, some staff members found their roles and responsibilities expanding without corresponding support structure expansion.

• Health systems should identify the concerns of both patients and providers through surveys, interviews, focus groups, and similar other efforts that will provide essential information for planning and directing resources effectively. For instance, surveys revealed that previous patients did not value the light housekeeping services that were provided under the old program. Thus, this difficult-to-administer service was replaced with more health care time and instruction from a qualified home health nurse. This approach also addressed the concerns of providers who wanted to ensure that the mother's and newborn's health needs could be met in the home. Physicians were invited to accompany nurses on their home health visits and were pleased to learn that proper care and testing were being provided adequately in the home.

PIPP has been an extremely valuable experience at HFHS. It has laid the groundwork for clinical process improvement efforts in a variety of other areas, including low back pain, breast care, chest pain and angina, depression, diabetes, and results reporting. It has provided a learning process used to develop infrastructure for other initiatives: a system-level physician champion, a public relations department to develop materials, and dedicated staff to roll out the improvement systemwide.

Based on the PIPP experience, new process initiatives will be system based and corporate directed. Local sites can still implement their own initiatives, but they must also comply with system initiatives.

As a testament to PIPP's success, the pediatric team intends to expand on PIPP's efforts. The next phase of PIPP is to implement an educational and clinical process for infants from birth through year two. All PIPP materials are being translated into Spanish and Arabic to reflect the composition of the system's patient population.

According to Deborah Ebers, vice president of business and labor relations, HFHS has not identified PIPP as a special program to employers. She explains, "We could take PIPP on a road show, but we tend to consider it a part of our overall maternity episode management. We also look for a period of stabilization before we use a program like PIPP for marketplace positioning."

* * * * * * *

### Mercy Health Services: Care Management Approach

The Care Management Strategy of Mercy Health Services (MHS), headquartered in Farmington Hills, Michigan, has evolved from prior work in clinical integration between 1994 and 1998. In 1997, the MHS Clinical Integration Priority Team drafted and approved a strategy planning and deployment model for fiscal years 1998 through 2000. The team's vision stated that MHS would develop a system of appropriate, effective clinical care that includes a seamless continuum of services, supports collaborative practice, and improves community health. The objectives were to:

- Improve clinical care through population health management.
- Expand the definition of the care continuum across care setting and the life cycle.
- Provide clinical input for clinical information systems development.
- Improve community health status.

After careful consideration, it was determined that this initiative should be transformed into the Care Management Strategy. The system has been challenged to develop an infrastructure that increasingly involves patients and families in clinical decision making, supports new methods of delivering care for populations, increases communication, and supports sharing of data across care sites. Barriers to accomplishing these objectives have included lack of clinical information systems to support the work and the challenge of obtaining clinicians' time as required. To date, initiatives have focused on obstetrical care, asthma care, community-acquired pneumonia, total hip replacement, and congestive heart failure. Accomplishments have included reducing length of stay by a full day for total joint replacement, decreasing length of stay for congestive heart failure patients from 5.7 to 5.1 days, and decreasing mortality from pneumonia while decreasing length of stay by one-half day.

## Current Initiative

MHS seeks to differentiate itself on the basis of measurable quality outcomes that result in "Exquisite Care Delivery" and "World Class Service" by providing care at the right place, time, and provider; coordinated care across the continuum; facilitated communication among providers, patients, and payers; promoting trusted, empowered, and teamwork behavioral changes; and accountability of senior management and clinical leadership. Care Management is an extension of MHS's past integration initiatives and seeks to improve clinical outcomes, become a preferred care delivery destination, improve customer loyalty, and become a stable and sustainable system.

MHS is now focusing its efforts on cardiovascular care, obstetrics, oncology, orthopedics, diabetes, and respiratory care. It plans to extend care management to clinical areas at the rate of one or two per year. The areas represent about 70 percent of the inpatient volumes. For each of the clinical areas, it has adopted three clinical outcome indicators to measure how well it is providing care for these patients. By design, only two of the twelve indicators require manual or alternative methods of data collection at the local site. All other indicators can be collected from existing databases. An example of the indicators being used is shown in Table 5.4.

The continuous measurement of clinical indicators is planned to create a tension for change and a willingness to explore new options in care delivery. Mercy expects significant variation in clinical outcomes across all MHS sites that will allow them to identify better practices that can be shared and replicated. The Care Management

Table 5.4. Care Management Indicators, Mercy Health Services.

| Indicator | Definition | Approved By | Likely Source | Frequency | Presentation |
|---|---|---|---|---|---|
| | Cardiovascular Disease | | | | |
| Number of hospital days/year/congestive heart failure patient (CHF) | Number of hospital days/year/CHF patient. CHF patients defined as patients with any of the following primary diagnosis codes: 402.01, 402.11, 402.91, 428.0, 428.8, and 428.9 | CLC | Jupiter | Monthly | Reported monthly: graphics and data. |
| ACE inhibitor use in CHF | (All CHF patients who are identified as being on an ACE inhibitor)/(CHF patient population) × 100%.  CHF patient population is defined as patients with any of the following primary diagnosis codes: 402.01, 402.11, 402.91, 428.0, 428.8, and 428.9. | CLC | Hospital reported | Monthly submission of data | Reported monthly: graphics and data. |
| Beta blocker use following AMI | To be determined as consistent as possible with public reporting methods | | Hospital reported | Monthly | Reported monthly: graphics and data. |

## Obstetrics/Gynecology

| | | | | | |
|---|---|---|---|---|---|
| Cesarean section rate | The number of women who delivered a baby(ies) by c-section divided by all deliveries.<br><br>(DRG370 + DRG371)/(DRG370 + DRG371 + DRG372 + DRG373 + DRG374 + DRG375) × 100% | MHS Quality Committee of the Board | Jupiter | Monthly | Reported monthly: graphics and data. |
| Vaginal birth after cesarean section rate | (DRG 372 through 375 with ICD-9 codes 654.20, 654.21, or 654.23)/(Sum of DRG 370 through 375 with ICD-9 codes 654.20, 654.21, or 654.23) × 100% | MHS Quality Committee of the Board | Jupiter | Monthly | Reported monthly: graphics and data. |
| Low birthweight babies (<2,500 g) | (Number of babies with ICD-9 codes 765.01-.08)/ (all babies delivered) × 100% | | Jupiter | Monthly | Reported monthly: graphics and data. |

## Orthopedics

| | | | | | |
|---|---|---|---|---|---|
| Total primary hip replacement average length of stay | Average length of stay for patients with a principal procedure code of 81.51 for patients not admitted through the ER. | CLC | Jupiter | Monthly | Reported monthly: graphics and data. |

Table 5.4. Care Management Indicators, Mercy Health Services, Cont'd.

| Indicator | Definition | Approved By | Likely Source | Frequency | Presentation |
|---|---|---|---|---|---|
| | Orthopedics | | | | |
| Total knee average length of stay | Average length of stay for patients with a principal procedure code of 81.54. Only knee replacement patients who were not admitted through the ER. | CLC | Jupiter | Monthly | Reported monthly: graphics and data. |
| Average number of complications of total hip replacement | Sum of all dislocations, postoperative infections, and thromboembolic events/number of THR patients | | Jupiter | Monthly | Reported monthly: graphics and data. |
| | Oncology | | | | |
| Breast cancer stage at diagnosis | Proportion of breast cancers diagnosed at each of stages I–IV | | Tumor Registry | Monthly | Reported monthly: graphics and data. |
| Average days of hospice care (inpatient and outpatient) | (Total days of hospice care at time of death)/(expired hospice patients) | | MCC database | Quarterly | Reported monthly: graphics and data. |
| Colon cancer stage at diagnosis | | | Tumor Registry | | |

*Source:* Mercy Health Services.

Initiative is envisioned to help MHS better coordinate existing initiatives, decrease duplication, increase shared learning, use resources more effectively, facilitate rapid replication of best practices, and ensure effective use of information services. It is built on clinical and physician integration principles that rely on clinical leaders to facilitate care management processes and goals.

MHS Clinical Quality is overseen by Bruce Van Cleave, executive vice president of MHS Professional Services. A detailed overview of the Care Management Initiative is shown in Figure 5.3. Among the critical success factors that MHS has identified to date in implementing its plans have been these:

- The importance of involving physicians from the beginning
- The need for strong information system support
- The need to evaluate and involve patients more actively in their care and in taking greater responsibility and authority
- Defining clear lines of responsibility and authority
- Emphasizing and focusing on quality indicators and outcome measures rather than cost

[Prepared with the assistance of Dr. Bruce Van Cleave and Louise Milobowski, R.N., M.S.N., at MHS.]

Figure 5.3. Overview of the Care Management Initiative,
Mercy Health Services.

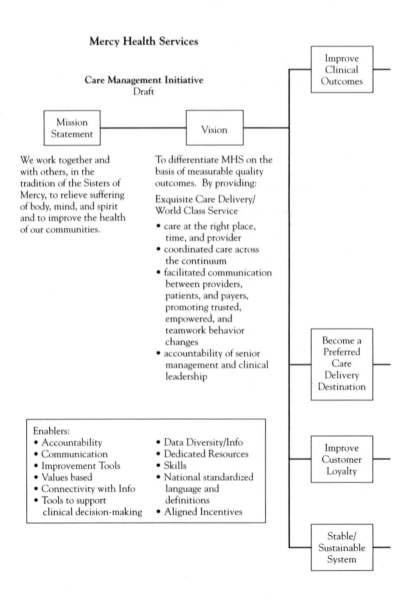

Reach/Exceed Targets:

| *Care Management Indicators:* | Target: |
|---|---|
| *Obstetrics* | |
| Cesarean Section Rate | 15% |
| Vaginal Birth after Cesarean Rate | 60% |
| Low Birth Weight Infant Rate | 5.0% |
| *Orthopedics* | |
| Hip Replacement (81.51) LOS | 3.65 days |
| Knee Replacement (81.54) LOS | 3.4 days |
| Complications of Hip Replacement | TBD |
| *Cardiovascular* | |
| ACE Inhibitor use in CHF | 70% |
| Beta Blocker use following AMI | 74% |
| Number of hosp days/yr/CHF pt | 11.0 days |
| *Oncology* | |
| Breast Cancer Stage at Diagnosis | TBD |
| Average Days of Hospice Care | TBD |
| Rectum & Colon Cancer Stage at Diagnosis | TBD |
| *Diabetes* | |
| Vascular complication rate | TBD |
| Hospital days/year | TBD |
| HgA1C | TBD |
| *Respiratory* | |
| Asthma 30 day readmit rate | TBD |
| Asthma ER visits/year/patient | TBD |
| Pneumonia mortality rate | TBD |

Locally driven indicators and targets (TBD)

---

Increased patient volumes in selected focus areas (outpatient + inpatient).

Decreased leakage of services to other facilities.

Indispensable to insurance carriers.

---

Proud to refer family and friends to MHS facilities/services.

Patient satisfaction tool indicates above average scores and/or a continual improvement from baseline.

---

Obtain 3–4% Operating Margin.

Effective and efficient use of clinical resources as reflected in profit versus loss for key clinical areas of focus.
[Net Revenue —Cost]

Figure 5.3. Overview of the Care Management Initiative, Mercy Health Services, Cont'd.

**Infrastructure and Reporting Capabilities:**
1. Design and implement CM model.
2. Develop infrastructure: communication plan, method(s) for data feedback, information system support, outcomes measurement, roles/accountability/people, approach to behavioral change management, knowledge and use of appropriate tools for process and practice variation, incentives alignment design.
3. Define care management core indicators, balancing indicators, and targets for each focus area.
4. Standardize outcomes measurement, reporting, and variance documentation (Governance/SMT/Medical Staff).
5. Complete pharmaceutical care reviews: pharmaceutical utilization, pharmacokinetics, and pharmacoeconomic guidelines.
6. Review financial data for reimbursement or contracting opportunities.
7. Review physician practice patterns monthly in comparison to peer group in focus areas.
8. Engage key physician and clinician champions to facilitate 1:1 communication with colleagues.
9. Create process to capture and report data beyond what is currently available in data warehouse (i.e., cost, across continuum, registry).
10. Expand data capabilities to include collection of: quality of life surveys, functional status, and customer satisfaction.
11. Create and disseminate "what if" scenarios" to assist with forecasting volumes, utilization patterns, and clinical variances.
12. Document ROI for care management/clinical improvement activities.

**Statewide Strategies: MHS Differentiation:**
13. Identify one to two focus areas based on the strongest clinical and financial opportunities for MHS.
14. Identify best practices in focus areas within MHS, set targets, and benchmark comparisons.
15. Link CHCS with each other to assist with improvement replication and rapid diffusion of information and innovation.
16. Convene MHS clinical network teams to address focus areas.
17. Standardize processes and/or products where appropriate within focus areas.
18. Effective "branding" of MHS services within the community.

**Locally Driven Initiatives:**
19. Identify one to three focus areas based on the strongest clinical and financial opportunities for the CHCS.
20. Identify best practices in focus areas within MHS and externally, set targets, and benchmark comparisons.
21. Convene local clinical network teams to address focus areas.
22. Link CHCS with each other to assist with improvement replication and rapid diffusion of information and innovation.
23. Implement nationally accepted scientific guidelines/algorithms for focus areas.
24. Standardize processes and/or products where appropriate within focus areas.
25. Implement complete customer satisfaction program.

**Evaluation and Planning:**
26. Evaluate FY 2000 work.
27. Create FY 2001 plan.

# 6

. . . . . . . . . . . . . . . . . . . . . . . . . . . . . . . . . .

# Governance and Management

In our earlier book, we noted that an organized delivery system stands on four pillars—its vision, culture, strategy, and leadership—that are either strengthened or weakened by the system's governance and management. Indeed, an effective governance and management structure will strengthen a system's performance. It will accomplish this by creating a clear vision for the organization, fostering a culture supportive of that vision, enabling the organization to implement its strategies, and providing the leadership necessary to guide ongoing change and ensure accountability to multiple stakeholders—patients, payers, regulators, the community, and others. But what makes for an effective governance and management structure at one organization will often be ineffective at another. Consequently, no standard, off-the-shelf governance or management structures (or models) universally apply to all organized delivery systems. Instead, "the framework on which your organization will be built must be flexible, inclusive, and farsighted" (Griffith, 1995, p. 12).

## Governance

The interdependent, collaborative nature of an ODS "limits the extent to which existing governance forms employed by stand-alone institutions or multi-hospital systems can be merely 'brought forward' or 'carried over'" (Pointer, Alexander, and Zuckerman, 1995, p. 4) to an ODS. Consequently, a significant challenge that organizations will face on their integration journey will be in designing the right governance and management model for their specific system (and market) at a given point in time. The optimal ODS governance and management structure must be sensitive to the organization's unique history, culture, and current structure (stage of evolution), as well as responsive to the specific characteristics of its market, including its likely speed of transformation.

Before an organization can create a structure that addresses its unique situation, it will have to reexamine the "theory of the business," based on the assumptions on which the organization has been built (Drucker, 1994). Organizations that continue to operate under the old theory, where the hospital (rather than the patient or consumer) is the center of the delivery system, will fail. Truly effective boards understand that one of their key roles is to create the future of the organization. This occurs through forward thinking, planning, and action. A considerable amount of the board's time must be spent deliberating and planning how the system will function in the future (Orlikoff, 1997). The organization must develop new assumptions about the environment, societal expectations, the market, the customer, and technology. It must also refine its specific mission and evaluate its core competencies and capabilities needed to achieve the mission. These assumptions must fit reality, and they must be consistent with each other, understood by all involved, and tested continuously.

Once these fundamental issues and future parameters have been defined, the organization must design governance and management structures that will facilitate the development and performance of a truly integrated company. To date, no single design has been adopted consistently by the more progressive integrated delivery systems around the country.

Instead, systems have experimented with every conceivable combination and permutation of governance and management structures. As a starting point, many systems have explored adaptations of governance models that seemed to work for traditional multihospital systems. Three of the more common governance structures under review are the centralized structure, with one systemwide governing board and no local governing boards with any legal or fiduciary authority; the decentralized structure, characterized by a systemwide corporate governing board and multiple boards at the operating unit level; and a modified centralized structure, which has a systemwide corporate governing board and a limited number of subsidiary boards (Morlock and Alexander, 1986).

To date, very few health care organizations have adopted a pure centralized governance structure, although one of our study participants, Sentara Healthcare, has had success with its centralized approach to governance. It abolished all operating unit boards and instead concentrated all governing responsibilities in a single board of the health system. Nevertheless, the decentralized model remains the most common, even among our study participants. For example, Advocate Health Care has adopted a modified centralized governance model. It has centralized most of its true governing activities with its system-level board, but has also retained governing councils at each of its operating units to oversee quality and maintain its connection to the local community. In contrast, Fairview Health System has pursued a truly decentralized approach to governance, believing strongly in the benefits gained by retaining true governance oversight at the local level. (See the case studies at the end of this chapter for more information on each of these systems.)

To select the preferred governance model available, an organization must decide how it will organize along four key dimensions:

- *Control.* First and foremost, an organization must determine whether it will be governed by a centralized or a decentralized board.

- *Structure.* If the organization adopts a decentralized structure, it will need to clarify how its subordinate boards should be used. Should a subordinate board be created for each operating unit, each region (if regions are necessary), or each group of operating units (for example, a subordinate board over the system's hospitals, long-term care facilities, medical groups, and so forth)? Some systems find that the most suitable structure requires a combination of these various options (for example, a board for each operating unit, which reports to a regional board, which then reports to the system board).

- *Functioning.* A system that has chosen to organize around multiple boards must clearly delineate the powers and authorities vested at each board level. Another option would be to have one "true" governing body at the system level and "advisory boards" at the institutional or regional levels. "An important caveat to remember is that form should follow function. A process that simply focuses on changing or streamlining the structure of governance without first addressing its function (especially the relative roles and responsibilities of multiple boards) is likely to cause more problems than it solves" (Orlikoff and Totten, 1996, p. 16).

- *Composition.* The organization must determine whether the overall system of governance will be representative or nonrepresentative. In representative boards, members are selected based on their relationship to a particular operating unit; with a nonrepresentative approach, elected members have no relationship to various components of the system. For example, a representative system would provide each operating unit with a seat on the parent board. The disadvantage of this type of system would be that as the system grows, the board will also grow, and it may reach an unmanageable size.

Furthermore, representative governance structures tend to impede system integration, because each board member often focuses on furthering the interests of his or her particular institution rather than striving to improve the position of the system overall. Organizations must also make a conscious effort to recruit board members with specific skill sets to serve on the board of an integrated delivery system (Pointer, Alexander and Zuckerman, 1995).

In sum, the governance model chosen should facilitate good governance, defined as the right people using the right facts to make the right decisions at the right time (Leatt and Leggatt, 1997).

## Management

In addition to governance models, ODSs are also experimenting with a wide range of management structures. Here too the optimal structure for each organization will be unique to the particular situation of that organization: the characteristics of its market, its history, its culture, and its vision and future goals. Regardless of the wide range of possible structures, however, ODSs will typically create management structures that are ordered around one of the following categories:

- Operating units (such as hospitals, physician practices, and long-term care organizations). A senior manager is named over each "division" of "like" organizations to establish common approaches to the delivery of care at that point along the care continuum.

- Geography. Market areas are typically subdivided along "natural" patient-consumer migration patterns—for example, broad regional or state lines or different areas of a metropolitan center. A senior manager is named to lead each "region" and typically is charged with the responsibility to facilitate the coordination of all health system activities operating in a common region.

- Functions (such as finance, strategy, nursing, and laboratory). A senior manager is assigned to lead the delivery of common functions across the system.

- Products and services (such as cardiac care, women's services, and imaging care). A senior manager is assigned to coordinate the delivery of "like" care across all appropriate operating units throughout the system.

There are as many variations on the management organizational structure as there are organized delivery systems. Like the implementation of particular governance models, management variations generally involve some type of hybrid of the approaches described. For example, it is common to organize different pieces of the system using different models. Often nonclinical support functions (such as finance, planning, and human resources) are organized at a system level, with perhaps site administrators for the function located at each operating unit. Coordination of clinical services (such as women's health and cardiac care) will generally involve matrix management with individuals "coordinating" activities from multiple operating units. Typically these individuals do not have line authority over either budgets or personnel for their areas of responsibility. Consequently, to be successful, these individuals must be extraordinary "influencers" of people.

It is essential that management structures be designed to be supportive of and consistent with the organization's approach to and structure for governance. "It does not make sense to have incompatible leadership structures, such as a system with decentralized governance and centralized management and clinical operations.

Compatible leadership structures facilitate efficient and effective system leadership" (Orlikoff, 1998, p. 14).

Central to the design of any particular structure is the determination of the system's internal goals. The specific organizational design flows from those decisions. Further, and perhaps more important, the best structure is also dependent on the unique skills, experiences, interests, and personalities of the people in the various leadership positions. What may seem reasonable and even desirable on paper can quickly pose difficulties if the individuals slated to sit in the various "boxes" do not possess the skills critical for success.

Furthermore, the size of the organization (in terms of geography of markets served and number of operating units or personnel) has an impact on possible options available to the system. Some divisions may be too big to run as a single division; others may be too diverse. Thus, the maturing ODS becomes an organization without walls—one whose management structure meets both internal and external (community) needs.

Finally, physician leaders are key to integration efforts, "reflecting the notion that physician-organization destinies are interdependent and inextricably intertwined" (Burns and Thorpe, 1993). Consequently, no matter how organizations structure their governance and senior management functions, physician leaders must play a critical leadership role. ODSs empower system physicians by allocating board seats (with voting rights) on all significant boards within the system. "Indeed, many of the recent changes in governance structure of integrated systems reflect an increasingly central role for physicians" (Alexander, Zuckerman, and Pointer, 1995, p. 73). Furthermore, physicians in senior management positions serve not only in staff and support roles (for example, as chief medical officer) but also have increasing line authority and responsibility embodied in their positions (for example, senior executive over physician practices and ambulatory services).

## Barriers and Challenges

Many systems have made progress in implementing more integrated delivery models since we wrote our first book, yet even today few seem to have successfully created a system of care that they would characterize as truly integrated. What makes this journey so difficult? From an overall management and governance perspective, we believe that six major barriers or challenges impede a system's integration efforts: (1) financial realities, (2) misunderstanding of the integration strategy, (3) historical roles and responsibilities, (4) shortage of talent with the right skills, (5) unwillingness to relinquish control, and (6) not bought into the strategy. An organization's governance, management, and aligned physicians must respond with strong leadership if the organization is to overcome these barriers.

### Financial Realities

Health care organizations across the country have seen significant decreases in profitability. Their reimbursement levels over the past few years have declined chiefly due to the implementation of the Balanced Budget Act, but other factors, such as managed care, employer coalitions, state Medicaid program changes, and related forces, have combined to make financing the delivery of care an ongoing challenge. In contrast, expenses continue to climb; the robust economy has created an all-time low in unemployment, pharmaceutical costs continue to soar, advancements in medical technology are real but translate into costly equipment, information systems needed to pull all the pieces together are outrageously expensive, and huge sums of cash were needed to address numerous Y2K issues. As a result, capital is scarce for most health systems. Many institutions abandoned their commitment to integration, believing that it was partly to blame for their financial woes. Others were easily diverted by various red-herring initiatives that appeared to be quick fixes to the critical situation at hand.

Regardless of the reaction, in an environment of financial crisis or other turbulence, whatever changes are appropriate for a particular organization, there is no question that board leadership must guide the way (Farrell, 1995). A focused and visionary leadership team is essential. Limited resources need not be an insurmountable barrier if management is able to prioritize efforts appropriately by designing truly effective governance and management structures that enable, rather than limit, the organization's performance.

## Misunderstanding of the Integration Strategy

Throughout the 1990s, health care organizations pursued a strategy of "integration" at an increasingly feverish pace. Seminars were held, articles written, and books read. Almost any health care leader asked could describe in great detail what an organized delivery system was, or at least should be. Everyone "knew" that the formation of that "desired" future state was critical to his or her future success. As a result, organizations by and large began the process of putting together the pieces—the "necessary" component parts for the system. Almost overnight, most of the nation's hospitals became a "system," whether their system was a single hospital with formally affiliated physicians or a multidimensional, multihospital system like our study participants. Regardless of size, the complexity of the organizations changed. With that change, the existing governance and management structures were inadequate to guide the organization in its new state.

As organizations struggled to modify governance and management structures to lead these newly formed organizations better, many forgot (or never really took the time initially to understand) what the "integration strategy" was all about. Some would say they were integrating to be prepared for managed care, specifically capitation, and perhaps that was why their system developed. However, from our perspective, the reason systems were developing was to begin to coordinate care for the patient. This would make it easier for the patient to receive the "right care at the right place at the right time." The intent was to improve quality of care and outcomes for patients. It should also give the providers the right information needed to deliver the appropriate care in a fashion that would be helpful to the patient; there would be no redundant testing or questioning to gather the same information multiple times. Instead, the organized delivery system would be a health care system truly created with the patient (or health care consumer) at the center.

Instead, traditional multihospital systems focused on models in which the assets of the facilities were controlled and owned through a common parent structure or a singular corporate model. These models have worked relatively well for horizontal integration, in which independent hospitals have combined with other hospitals to form systems. However, the success of an organized delivery system will be characterized by the degree to which it creates a seamless continuum of care that links organizations at different stages of the health care delivery process. This effort drives systems to adopt a vertical, rather than horizontal, integration strategy.

Because completely closed systems are not generally accepted—Americans demand choice—a vertical integration strategy will be flawed if it predicates organizational success on common control and ownership of all parts of the system. A more appropriate implementation of the vertical integration strategy is to ensure that virtual integration, or what we call *behavioral* integration, occurs through implementing effective contractual relationships (Goldsmith, 1994). Successful contractual relationships must include quality standards and the ability to monitor not just the outputs but also quality and outcomes. Developing information technologies, including Web-based technologies with their relatively low expenses and open standards, will further individual providers' ability to develop virtual integration relationships.

The experience of the study systems also suggests that two other "V's" are important to implementing a vertical integration strategy. The first of these is that vertically integrated organizations must reflect *visual integration*. In other words, the consumer must perceive and experience the products and services produced by the organized delivery system as being seamless. Organized delivery systems that effectively meet the challenges of the new health care environment will have holographic qualities. When an organized delivery system behaves like a hologram, visual integration is achieved.

The second "V" can best be described as *visceral integration*, or the degree to which the partners in a vertically integrated relationship regard the system's success as of significant importance. The partners must have an emotional and financial commitment to the strategy, not merely an intellectual commitment to it. The key distinction is the ability to commit financial and human resources to the strategy so that its partners will feel pain if the system is not successful in reaching its goals. As one system executive described this level of commitment, "It is a time in which we cannot have deep pockets and short arms." System leaders must be willing to commit appropriate resources to the vertical integration strategy and then implement and manage it aggressively.

Unfortunately, many managers and clinicians have not yet internalized this strategy. Conceptually, most agree with it, but many have yet to be convinced that building a system around the health care consumer will be viable. Without true understanding of or commitment to the strategy, it will be impossible to achieve.

### Historical Roles and Responsibilities

Shedding the weight of the past is unquestionably one of the most difficult challenges organizations have attempted to resolve over the past few years. Most continue to struggle with it. All systems, structures, personnel, and reward mechanisms have been designed to support a model of care very different from that required of tomorrow's successful providers. Systems have started realigning incentives, but most admit they have not yet completed the task. In the past, the focus was on treating illness, caring for the individual, and filling schedules and beds by increasing visits and admissions. In this world, the hospital was king, and all governance and management activities supported that reign. As a result, "it is time to pay due respect to the past—perhaps even grieve over it—but then to get on with inventing and managing the new delivery systems to meet the needs of the future" (Shortell and others, 1993, pp. 452–453).

The new health care organization will be responsible for a very different set of activities. It must focus on maintaining wellness; provide access to a continuum of care and services that are "value added"; deliver care in the most cost-effective manner and in the most appropriate location; manage a network of services that it likely will not own; and actively manage quality. Since the rush to integration began, most hospital-based health care delivery systems have been assembling the "pieces to prepare for their new responsibilities. However, their focus has been on filling in their continuums of care through strategic alliances or outright acquisitions rather than on developing the necessary infrastructure to make the pieces work well together. In particular, many systems are collapsing structures to force a "desegregation" and, they hope, an integration of their operating units. However, it is important to note that integration and desegregation are not the same. Integration and centralization are also very different concepts. Integration requires an interactive, interdependent relationship to be formed among the various "integrated" entities. Simply aggregating a system's operating units into a common reporting structure will not create a seamless, well-coordinated health care system. These distinctions are critical and, if understood, will help an organization revise various roles and responsibilities throughout the system to facilitate and support the desired change.

Many ODSs have invested a great deal of effort in integrating their operating units over the past four years. The major focus, however, has been on financial and legal relationships among the various entities. So far, most patient care delivery systems and most patients have not seen significant operating change. Integrating clinical systems and operations remains the challenge for the next decade.

In the past, governing bodies were dominated by hospital issues, hospital people, and an interest in continuing to spend resources on the creation of a facility-rich empire. Board structures generally were decentralized and cumbersome, often reflecting a variation of the decentralized governance structure. Each operating unit generally had its own board, and as long as that unit performed within the agreed-on financial parameters and did not pursue activities that conflicted with the system, the board was free to pursue whatever strategy it chose for its market.

In the future, governance of the health system (whether it involves multiple boards or not) must support the *system's* goals, and if multiple boards are maintained, each must ensure that its operating unit contributes to the system's future success. Furthermore, all boards within the system will need to monitor different measures to assess performance—of the system overall, of the operating unit, and of the senior management team. For example, traditional accounting and financial controls should be supplemented by additional focus on more balanced performance scorecards, using measures such as customer satisfaction, quality outcomes, market demand, and community health status.

The complex and duplicative board structures that evolved in health care institutions resulted from attempts to solicit adequate representation from key community leaders—although community representation within these structures largely meant input and guidance primarily from the *business* community. Rarely was there more than token representation from physicians, public health, and other health-related executives on a system board. In the future, the governing structures of more advanced health care systems will reflect their organizations' commitment to community health with a diversified board whose members understand the delivery of services at different points along the care continuum.

From a manager's perspective, meeting expectations from a wide constituency remains a juggling act. Daily challenges grow in difficulty. Financial pressures have continually intensified and show no signs of abating. Finding and managing employees has become more difficult in almost universally tight labor markets and America's increasingly multicultural society. Competition for patients and other customers and resources intensifies by the year. Meanwhile, successful managers are expected to position their departments, facilities, and institutions for a highly uncertain future. In the past, they would strive to build their organization's market image and reputation to increase inpatient volumes and demand for high-tech (and high-cost) outpatient services. They focused their efforts on wooing the physician, with little regard to the health care consumer.

The new world that health care managers face today is remarkably different from the one they faced just a few years ago. E-commerce is rapidly reshaping the competitive landscape for purchasing services ranging from pharmaceuticals to medical supplies to online medical advice. Real-time health and medical information is easily accessible and is readily available from a multitude of sources; as a result, consumers have become more informed and discriminating purchasers. The Internet and its capabilities are allowing long-distance medical care to widen the reach of providers. Adapting to the competitive landscape and the rapidly changing environment only exacerbates the challenges that health care managers face while pushing their organizations toward integration.

Many managers who have been successful in the past do not understand how they can succeed in this new environment. They may understand in theory where their new emphasis should be, but many lack the experience or knowledge base to run some of the growing segments of the new health care delivery system's business. Managing in the new health care system requires a new set of skills that go beyond simply managing new types of patient care or administrative activity. Today's and tomorrow's managers must manage virtual networks. They must manage change itself, guiding their employees and their systems through future shifts. Tomorrow's managers must understand not only how the new health care system works and their role within it, but also how to apply a new set of measures to determine success.

Without informed and enlightened leadership, the management team of the past may unintentionally restrict the growth of these new critical activities by allocating too many resources to outdated services rather than to an expanded continuum of care. This inclination is particularly true of the system cash cow, which is "usually the flagship of the system and, as such, has often been granted the most autonomy to pursue its own interests" (Shortell and others, 1993, p. 453). What will be imperative for each management team (and governing body) to understand is that "today's 'cash cows' may well become tomorrow's 'dogs,' and continued investment in them to the exclusion of newly emerging priorities could bring down the entire system" (Shortell and others, 1993, p. 453).

Finally, to facilitate the transition, new or evolving systems must clearly define the new roles and responsibilities of board members and managers, including physicians. Part of the difficulty in accomplishing change today is that key organizational leaders do not precisely understand how they will fit into the system or where they should direct their attention. It has been said that people pay attention to those activities for which they are rewarded. To encourage new behaviors in the system's key leadership, in particular its management, the reward structure must change. If managers are told to be creative and to take risks, for example, they should no longer remain subject to outmoded performance evaluation systems or inappropriate financial hurdles.

One system in the study significantly altered its incentive compensation program to reflect its new system goals. This innovative program has both short- and long-term incentives. All employees in the organization are eligible to receive an annual bonus payment based on several factors, the key being financial performance. A threshold operating margin percentage must be reached for the program to take effect; once this has been reached, other variables enter into the equation. The incentive program is equally based on system and divisional results, which has driven integration across business units and systemwide focus on financial performance. In sum, board members and managers should be encouraged to support new business practices with incentives that hold them accountable for their actions through a meaningful relationship between risk and reward.

Finally, one cannot overstate the importance of managing the pace of the change. It may have felt that change occurred quickly in the past, but it is increasing its pace at an exponential rate. Today's Internet-familiar consumer finds a minute delay for service almost unbearable. As a result, significant change is inevitable; however, moving an organization too far too fast can be just as disabling as not moving it at all. Consequently, as an organization considers various governance and management models, it should assess in what form and at what speed the market will change, and pursue the new structure with a level of intensity in keeping with that organization's readiness for change.

### Shortage of Talent with the "Right" Skills

From a governance perspective, many board members bring a wide variety of backgrounds to their roles as a trustee: "Altruism, skills in their business or professional areas, connections with important constituencies, and concern for the needs addressed by the organization" (Kovner, Ritvo, and Holland, 1997, p. 88). Unfortunately, these skills do not represent a comprehensive set of characteristics for performing effectively as a trustee. Some of the more notable core skills necessary are "monitoring and assessing organizational performance, translating values into clear statements of guiding mission and objectives, setting priorities, and shaping the organization's future directions in a complex environment" (Kovner, Ritvo, and Holland, 1997, p. 89). Core skills necessary to succeed as an effective trustee may not have been communicated to the potential member prior to his or her nomination or evaluated or even considered when appointed to the board. As a result, many trustees are unprepared for the demands of governing a highly complex, sophisticated organization, such as today's organized delivery system.

Organizations often have difficulty implementing their integration plans not because the plan stems from an incorrect strategy but because managers do not understand the strategy, disagree with it, lack sufficient incentives to motivate action, or lack sufficient skills to implement it. As with so many other of these critical hurdles, the skills needed to succeed in the past are not the same skills needed to succeed in the future. Many administrators who grew up in hospitals are uncertain about their new roles and do not fully comprehend the relationship of hospitals, physician partners, other continuum services, payers, managed care products, and communities. If an integrated system is to work, managers must thoroughly understand these relationships. Otherwise they may feel like targets of change rather than agents of change, and they may fear (potentially with some reason) that their power and influence are being reduced.

Once the appropriate governance and management models have been selected, individuals will determine how well the infrastructure works. Unfortunately, many of the key system board members and executives have never had to think "system" as opposed to "operating unit," and consequently they may not be as skilled in the new world as they were in the old. Many leaders do not even know what other system operating units do or how they contribute to the overall system strategy, which means these leaders will have particular difficulty integrating the units. Furthermore, an essential source of key leadership talent is the organization's physicians. Unfortunately, like managers, few physicians have the right skills to allow them to succeed in leadership roles—including "people" skills, analytical ability, business acumen, and "big picture" vision—while also commanding respect among other physicians and staff. Physicians with an appropriate blend of these capabilities are in high demand and difficult to recruit. Consequently, organizations must carefully select and groom potential physician leaders so that a pool of candidates will be available to the organization over the long term.

### Unwillingness to Relinquish Control

Historically, boards, managers, and physicians have each retained some degree of autonomy and control. Today, as the discussion turns to integration and collaboration, health care leaders are not sure what will happen if they give up control. Although distributing control among a variety of leaders and functions can be difficult, studies show that organizations willing to do so seem to function better in changing environments.

The research shows that both group and developmental cultures can foster an environment that supports integration. Specifically, a group culture—characterized by an emphasis on flexibility and trust, a participatory leadership style, and sensitivity to many viewpoints during decision making—supports integration. Similarly, a developmental culture—identified by an emphasis on flexibility, an entrepreneurial and risk-taking leadership style, and empowerment at all levels to facilitate quick decision making—also supports integration. Furthermore, empowerment alone promotes an organization's *transactive memory*, defined as employee and member knowledge of what each other knows (Wegner, 1986). The greater an organization's transactive memory is, the greater is its ability to diffuse learning throughout the organization and to adapt to a rapidly changing environment (Argote, 1993).

The only way an organization will ever be able to respond quickly to a rapidly changing environment is to loosen the "control belt." Indeed, if one looks at the winners of the Malcolm Baldrige Award (which recognizes organizations nationwide for the quality of their products and services), a hallmark of the leaders of these organizations is their willingness to empower both personnel and partners to serve their customers best. Similarly, a recent case study of ten systems notes that "almost without exception, in the process of becoming a more integrated system, hospital administrators and boards have relinquished a significant share of their authority" (Coddington, Moore, and Fischer, 1994, p. 117).

## Not Bought into the Strategy

Another key challenge that leaders must address is engaging all levels of the organization to buy in to the integration strategy. Leaders must develop a comprehensive approach to engage each different category of employee, from front-line service providers, to managers, to clinicians, to trustees. Because incentives for each group are dramatically different, managers must tailor their approaches accordingly.

Over the years, many organizations have enjoyed long traditions of success as a result of their ability to develop and perfect certain characteristics and behaviors. However, when the environment changes and a new set of parameters for success is defined, different factors will determine organizations' relative competitive positions. Past success is no longer a valid predictor of future success; in fact, it may be a predictor of future failure.

Some organizations have attempted to implement change and suffered setbacks or failure. This only reinforces the desire to return to behaviors that produced success in the old health care market. These old behaviors may bring limited success for a time, but the market will pass such organizations by, and the need to change will ultimately reappear. Furthermore, organizations that start down the path to integration recognize that "overcoming cultural and organizational barriers will require the support of governance, an external push from the environment, and good luck in the process" (Hunt, 1996, p. 50).

Thus, painful though it may be, organizations must replace the familiar and the comfortable with the unproved. How they cope will vary. In a world of tremendous change, taking a giant leap of faith based only on a "trust us" rationale results in an exceedingly justifiable fear of failure and a real skepticism around the strategy itself. Organizations must both acknowledge that skepticism and seek to root it out. How successful they are will affect their long-term success.

## Key Success Factors

In the future, providing high-quality health services at competitive costs will be critical, and organizations will not be capable of achieving this goal "with outmoded organizational systems and processes" (Griffith, 1995, p. 12). Analyses of study participants suggest that the following actions can help an organization build the structures it needs to help break down internal barriers and ensure success: streamline governance structures and processes, redefine management roles, develop strong physician leaders, and implement broader performance accountability criteria.

### Streamline Governance Structures and Processes

Some suggest that "because of the unique position of boards, governance is potentially the ultimate integrator" (Pointer, Alexander, and Zuckerman, 1995, p. 3). Indeed, in regard to policy and strategy, the board level is the only place within the system where every piece finally comes together. However, in a fast-paced world, organizations no longer have the luxury of time to evaluate, debate, analyze again, build consensus, and then decide which strategic move makes the most sense. Instead the key is focus: getting the right information to the right people at the right time to make a decision. How well a board is able to "mobilize and focus their resources on key strategic priorities" (Kovner, Ritvo, and Holland, 1997, p. 88) will contribute to its overall effectiveness.

One of the more significant dimensions that affect governance processes is its structure. As organizations become more integrated, multiple board structures appear to complicate the process of governing. Especially where operating units serve a common marketplace, maintaining a segregated, dispersed system of governing may be counterproductive. Some systems (like Sentara Healthcare, described in the case study at the end of this chapter) have found it most effective to collapse all boards into a single governing body charged with the governance of the entire organization. Others (like

Advocate Health Care, also profiled in a case study at the end of this chapter) also have collapsed the main policy-setting responsibilities for the system to the health system board; however, to maintain significant ties to the many communities it serves, they have created governing councils at each of their operating units that monitor local quality-of-care issues. Organizations that serve several distinct regions also continue to streamline their governance processes, but they do so by region. One added benefit to having multiple governing bodies within a single system is they can serve as a fertile source for developing future board members for the main system board. By creating streamlined governance processes and structures, the organization will be nimble enough to respond to whatever new competitive threat or internal issue emerges.

### Redefine Management Roles

Management practices and skills of the past are not necessarily the best skills for the future. As with governance, management must be streamlined so that the decision-making process is quick and its organizational structure is nimble enough to respond rapidly to the market dynamics. Most of the study participants experienced numerous management reorganizations throughout the study. These changes typically involved combining the management of functions and services across the delivery system—essentially breaking down historical barriers and "smokestacks." Often a single individual was appointed as regional manager, responsible for the entire continuum of care within a defined geographic area. Many positions were eliminated and individuals reassigned to a wide variety of responsibilities. These efforts generally included integrating all types of care (inpatient and outpatient acute care, primary care, rehabilitative care, and so on) and support functions (human resources, information management, TQM, and managed care) in a coordinated fashion at the system level. Systems outside our study have taken similar action.

As a result of this continuous change, critical to any system's future success will be the presence of strong leadership. Leadership must be capable of clearly communicating change—explaining not only the rationale behind the change but also creating a burning platform to motivate the desired change. The leader of the new system must also clarify for management and others what their role will be in the new system: how they will personally contribute to the achievement of the vision. This should apply to both senior management and front-line employees.

Finally, systems must restructure the reward system to provide incentives for important activities and penalties for those that are counterproductive. Many of the study participants' senior managers are rewarded based on overall *system* performance (such as cost reductions, financial results, patient satisfaction, enrollment growth, and system market share), and no longer on the bottom-line performance of their operating unit alone (this latter incentive fosters counterproductive competition among system units). ODSs need their managers to focus on the competition outside the system, not within it.

### Develop Strong Physician Leaders

Physician leadership is required at the board level, within the senior management team, and within affiliated physician group practices. Systems must identify physician champions who can set direction, provide them with the necessary authority and support to succeed, and adequately reward them for their contributions. (See Chapter Four for additional discussion of this topic.)

### Implement Broader Performance Accountability Criteria

As systems become more attentive to the health of local consumers and ultimately share in responsibility for the health of the community, they will need to develop broader performance accountability criteria. These criteria should address access, cost, quality, and outcome measures regarding the needs of multiple external stakeholder groups, including patients, employers, payers, community groups, regulators, and accreditation bodies, among others. At the same time, systems must develop measures that are useful for internal stakeholders, including physicians, nurses, other health professionals, executives, and board members. Such measures become the raw material for use in report cards and, perhaps more important, the input for interactive control systems (Simons, 1995) that enable organized delivery systems to take corrective action and initiate continuous improvement efforts. Some have referred to these measures as developing instrument panels that enable organized delivery systems to manage wisely, much as the cockpit crew on an airplane needs instrument panels to fly safely (Nelson and others, 1995).

The approach is similar to the "balanced scorecard" approach adopted by a number of corporations in other fields (Kaplan and Norton, 1992, 1993). Alexander, Zuckerman, and Pointer (1995) conclude that broadly based, balanced scorecards help both management and governance evaluate the extent to which the system gains advantages and adds value through integration strategies. Examples include measures of customer service and satisfaction, quality and outcome of clinical processes, cost and financial performance, growth, and degree of system integration. Figures 6.1 through 6.3 provide examples of balanced scorecards that the Henry Ford Health System (HFHS) uses to measure performance.

Henry Ford Health System also uses this methodology to track performance on other measures of system performance. The quality indicators scorecard (Figure 6.2) measures performance across three broad categories: chronic care, prevention, and acute care. The customer satisfaction scorecard (Figure 6.3) measures satisfaction across the continuum of services HFHS provides. Data for these measures are drawn from both internal HFHS-developed satisfaction measurement tools and nationally administered patient satisfaction measures, including these:

- Inpatient care satisfaction

- Outpatient care satisfaction

- Henry Ford Medical Group access satisfaction

- Behavioral care satisfaction

Figure 6.1. Operational Performance Indicators Scorecard, Henry Ford Health System.

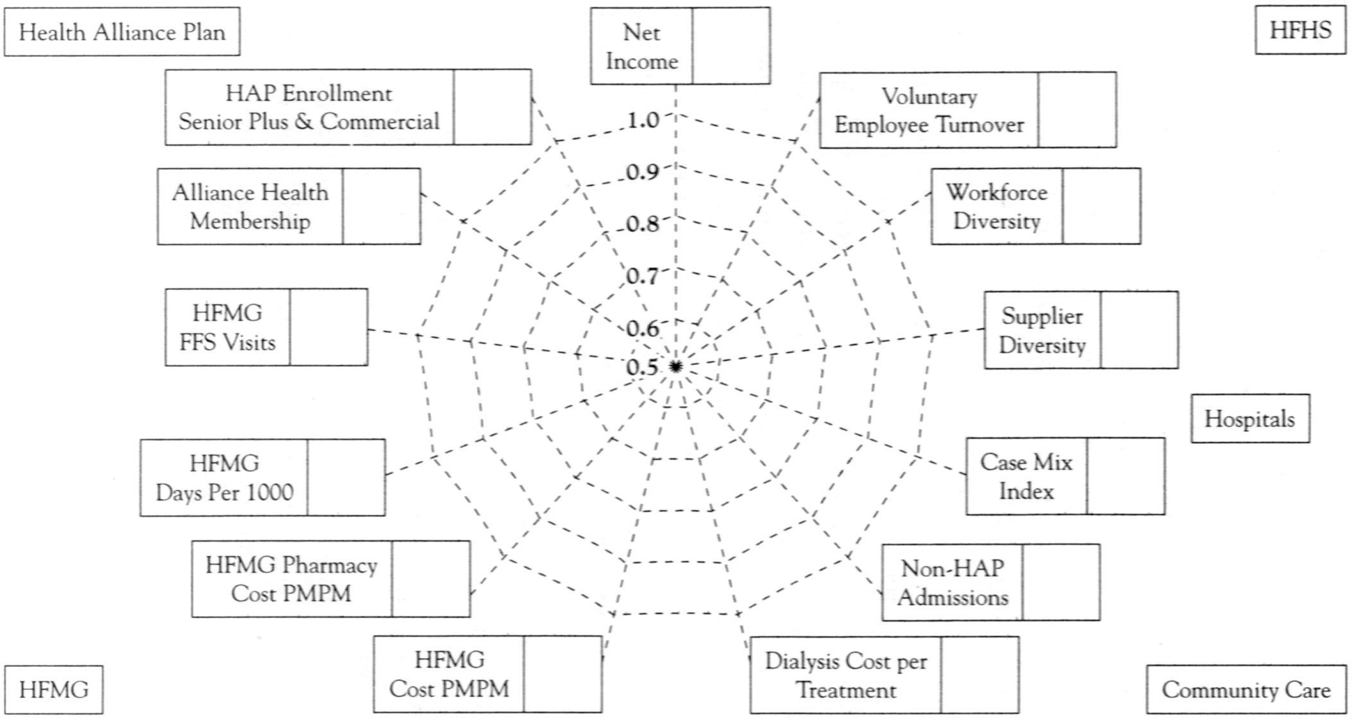

Figure 6.2. Quality Indicators Scorecard, Henry Ford Health System.

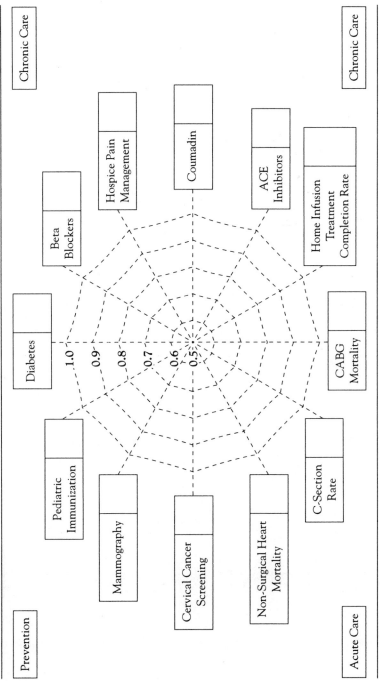

Figure 6.3. Customer Satisfaction Indicators Scorecard, Henry Ford Health System.

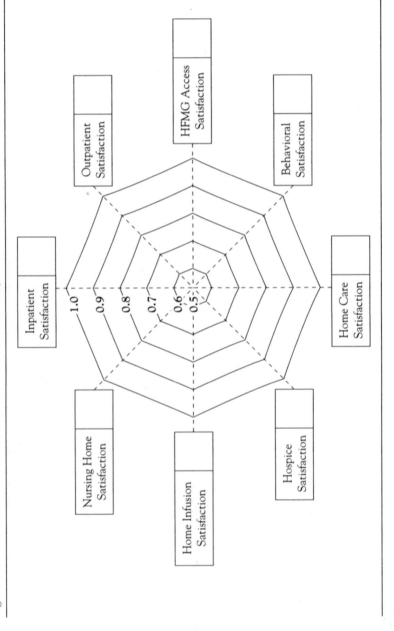

- Home care satisfaction

- Hospice satisfaction

- Home infusion satisfaction

- Nursing home satisfaction

Figure 6.4 shows some of the Mercy Health System's planned measures, which are directly linked to the system's strategic objectives and goals.

The strength of these performance measurement systems lies in their ability to provide incentives to caregivers, executives, and board members to monitor elements that truly make a difference to the organization's competitive position, while also providing key information useful to external bodies.

## Future Challenges

Most systems today are still focusing their efforts on assembling the right pieces. Eventually, however, they will need to determine how to make these pieces work together effectively. The critical choice at that point will be selecting the preferred model of integration, along with the governance and management structures that serve as fundamental building blocks for creating value for patients and purchasers alike.

Whichever model is pursued, the central goal is to strike a balance among an ODS's three key constituents: physicians, institutional providers (hospitals, home health agencies, long-term care facilities, ambulatory care settings, and so on), and payers. In successful systems, these elements maintain equilibrium through aligned or common governance, management, and financial incentives that reward the players for appropriately matching medical resources with the needs of payers and patients (Bartling, 1995).

Figure 6.4. Planning and Deployment Framework for Mercy Health Services, Fiscal Year 1998–2000 Strategic Plan.

MISSION  All of the Strategies Within This MHS Strategic Plan Will Be Undertaken to Increase the Long-Term Effectiveness of Mercy Health Services in Advancing the Healing Ministry of Jesus into the 21st Century. As This Plan Is Implemented, a System-Wide Dialogue Will Be Completed to Discern Additional Opportunities for Better Understanding and Integrating Our Mission and Values in the Face of a Changing Healthcare Environment.

FY 98-2000 STRATEGIC OBJECTIVES

**Community Partnerships**

1. Continuously Improve Community Health Through Community Partnerships and Advocacy, Focusing on Populations-at-Risk[a]

**Growth**

2. Increase Patients Served and Committed Lives as a System and in Each CHCS Service Area

**Quality/Value**

3. Continuously Improve Quality of Care and Service, Meeting or Exceeding Patient/Client Requirements

4. Effectively Integrate Services Across the Care Continuum and in Partnership With Our Physicians

5. Continuously Reduce Costs to Provide Best Value

6. Continuously Improve the Capability, Adaptability, and Quality of Work Life of Our Employees

FY 98-2000 VISION

Mercy Health Services Will Continue to Build One of the Country's Outstanding Integrated Catholic Healthcare Systems

We Will Meet or Exceed the Requirements of Our Patients and Other Clients by Continuously Improving Our Quality and Value to the Highest Benchmark Standards

We Will Use Our System's Growing Strength to Improve Community Health and to Serve and Advocate for Populations-at-Risk

VALUES

• Mercy

• Human Dignity

• Justice

• Service

• Preferential Option for the Poor

[a]Special commitment to the poor and to issues affecting women and children.

Two approaches commonly employed to achieve this balance are to include leaders from each of these key system components on the senior management team of the system and to create incentives for each leader that encourage cooperation—rather than competition—among the various divisions. Sentara, for example, has no significant meetings among its management team members without representatives from both its health plan and provider divisions present.

Another key strategic challenge that ODSs will face will be to amass the appropriate talent to succeed. In particular, leaders and managers in this new world of health care will require a radically different skill set from that of their predecessors. Some of these "new world" skills include systems thinking, negotiation, conflict management, change management, CQI, team building, and network and relationship management. Furthermore, the leader must be an implementer, not just a visionary.

Implementing systems of care that promote integration across the continuum also requires capital. In the future, the capital for such system development will come less from the operating margins of the system and more from strategic alliances and partnerships with others. Some of those alliances may involve totally new relationships among suppliers—biotech companies, device companies, and pharmaceutical companies, for example—and delivery systems, particularly given that the former have significant sums of capital available relative to the latter.

Systems must also encourage experimentation at all levels. The new "business" of health care must be almost continually reinvented, particularly when one's objectives have been achieved, rapid growth prevails, and one's own organization or one's collaborators and competitors experience unexpected success or failure (Drucker, 1994). ODSs of the future will have neither the luxury to establish fixed rules nor the time to evaluate each move systematically. An organization may establish parameters, but all personnel should have the flexibility, authority, and empowerment to respond quickly to situations as they arise. The organization will benefit from experimenting, learning, and experimenting some more to improve service quality continuously. An ODS's governance and management structures and its physician leadership must promote and support such behavior.

Finally, many systems are beginning to realize that each governance or management model presents a series of trade-offs, and the decisions associated with choosing one can be tremendously difficult and pose serious consequences. What are the short-term political costs of implementing various models? What are the ramifications for the organization if a particular model is not implemented? What is the best timing to implement a change? Must it happen today, or can it wait? Will a given model provide room for future growth and change? Most important, does the management and governance structure support the clinical caregiving process? If not, the net result may be structures whose components are not truly integrated and thus cannot work together.

### Advocate Health Care

Advocate Health Care is a not-for-profit, faith-based health care organization based in Oak Brook, Illinois. It was formed in January 1995 as the merger of EHS Health Care and Lutheran General HealthSystem. Since the merger, Advocate has transformed itself into one of the leading integrated delivery systems in the country. In 1999, SMG Marketing Group ranked it number one on the list of the nation's Top 100 Integrated Healthcare Networks.

Advocate has pursued an aggressive strategy of integration of both its governance and management functions. Its first strategic plan was developed during late 1995 and early 1996 by a team of board members, executive management, and physician leadership. "An extensive planning process was designed to maximize participation, encourage rigorous analysis, develop common beliefs about the nature of the future environment and to commit to a course of action for the fulfillment of Advocate's mission, values and philosophy" (Advocate Health Care, 1999, p. 1). The strategic vision of the organization was to create a well-coordinated, truly integrated health care system—one that results in improved outcomes for the patients under its care. For Advocate, integration was not simply an outcome itself, but a means to achieving its real goal: improved performance. Accordingly, Advocate leadership has closely followed this plan, committed to achieving the goals outlined at the organization's inception.

## Governance

The merger of EHS and Lutheran General HealthSystem into Advocate brought together two contrasting governance models. In an effort to integrate from the top down, a consolidated corporate governance structure was put into place that created one system-level board (see Figure 6.5). Advocate chose the single structure governance model for a number of key reasons. First, senior leadership believed that integration throughout the remainder of the organization could not occur without a strong example set by the most senior levels of the organization. Second, in the rapidly changing Chicago market, Advocate needed to be flexible enough to respond quickly to market dynamics, and third, to take advantage of Advocate's size and power in the market, a consistent and unified message from the governing board needed to be heard.

The new system board consists of twenty-one members, including four physicians and three ex officio members. Initially, each church sponsor elected half of the members to the combined system board. As a result, it was very apparent which board members had been elected by which sponsor in the early stages of governance development. However, as the governance structure and function became clearer and a level of trust was established among members, barriers were eliminated, and the focus moved to governing the new organization.

The single structure governance model has been highly beneficial in helping Advocate to react quickly to changes in the Chicago market. The board's broad and diversified membership and perspective have been key in Advocate's ability to streamline decision

Figure 6.5. Governance Structure, Advocate Health Care.

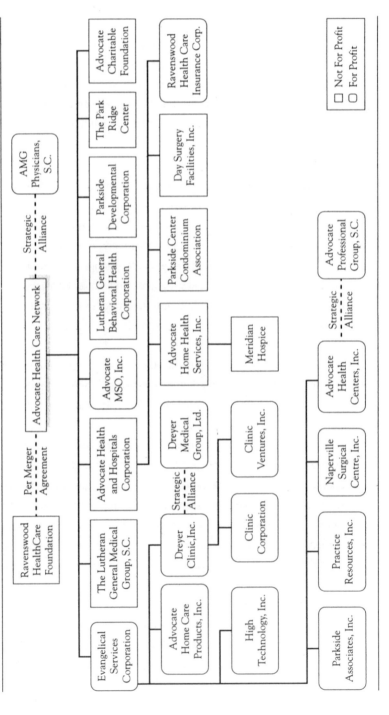

making and facilitate the development of an integrated system. In addition, board members serve on the operating unit governing councils as ex officio members by virtue of being directors of the Advocate Health Care Board. This helps the system board to be more closely aligned with the issues that Advocate's local operating units face.

Although Advocate was committed to having a streamlined governance structure, it also recognized the value of retaining a close tie to its many communities through some kind of governing vehicle at each operating unit. Consequently, rather than burdening the system with multiple policy-setting bodies that must be actively managed and involved in redundant decision-making processes, Advocate created governing councils at each of its operating units.

They look like a board, in that their membership comprises key stakeholders from that operating unit's community; however, their functions are focused on quality management, community relations, and implementation of the system strategies at their institution. Some of their more notable charges include providing input into the strategic planning and budgeting processes, as well as oversight for credentialing processes. All operating unit–level governing councils are accountable to the system board.

There have been some challenges in implementing the new governance model at the operating unit level. As a result of the power and authority given to the system board, operating unit governing councils have sometimes had difficulty understanding their role and responsibility to the organization. Management has taken steps to clarify both an internal role in assisting management and an external role developing relationships in the community. Furthermore, it is management's intention for the governing council position to serve as a training ground for future members of the system board. However, with its "nonpolicy setting" role and sizable commitment of time (six board meetings, two committee meetings, and two retreats annually), attracting members to the governing councils may be difficult.

Advocate has placed a large emphasis on governance development activities in an effort to educate and integrate the governance function across the system. These activities are a critical tool in preparing governing council members for potential seats at the system board in the future. Board members also participate in an annual assessment of governance performance. Members assess both individual and collective performance and provide management with their perspective on gaps in the governance process. This assessment provides management with key information to improve processes and identify characteristics for new trustees to be addressed in the nomination process.

To date, Advocate believes that its governance structure has realized many of the benefits the architects of the system anticipated. Leadership was able to push integration strategies from the top down, and it has been able to react quickly to changes in the market to take advantage of opportunities for continued integration and growth. Management has also been pleased with the willingness of its board and governing council members to serve in capacities throughout the organization and function as a positive liaison to the communities that Advocate serves.

Management continues to be pleased with the design and functionality of its governance system. Through consistent efforts at integrating board membership, developing appropriate roles within the organization and externally in the community, and providing governance development activities, Advocate has developed a well-run, highly integrated governance function. Annual assessment by board members and management, it hopes, will improve its model of governance.

## Management

Advocate was created as a result of the merger between EHS and Lutheran General HealthSystem. Together, they represented a very large organization with operating units covering a wide geographic area. As a result, there was a strong belief at its inception that the best way to manage this new organization would be to divide it into regions. A regional structure could enable management to decentralize where appropriate, stay closer to the customer, and provide managers with a greater sense of empowerment within their region. Consequently, the greater Chicago metropolitan area was divided into three geographic regions, each with an executive vice president who was accountable for the performance of all operating units within the area. Unfortunately, the regional executives became advocates for the sites within the region instead of a source of continuity across facilities and a catalyst for systemwide integration. Furthermore, the structure itself added an extra, and an expensive, layer of management onto the new organization.

After two years of the regional leadership model, Advocate disbanded it in favor of a new model led jointly by an executive vice president of operations and an executive vice president who was also the chief medical officer. The regional leadership positions were eliminated, and all of the operating unit management were placed under one of these two leaders. This remains the structure (see Figure 6.6). Experience to date has led management to conclude that integration is significantly further along as a result of the change.

In retrospect, Advocate CEO Richard Risk noted, "I think [the regional structure] actually caused the organization not to integrate as fast as it could have." Several variables contributed to the decision to eliminate the regional management model at Advocate. Key among these was the additional layer of management added to Advocate's structure, which provided some pockets of operating efficiency but ended up being more bureaucratic and expensive in the long run. Another variable was the internal competition and the disconnection that operating units felt from corporate leadership. The regional-level management was a barrier as the newly merged organizations attempted to integrate operations, structures, systems, and cultures. Advocate management noted that it did not believe that the regional organization structure model was inherently flawed, but thought that in its experience, the model did not enable it to optimize its integration strategies. Ultimately it was not the right structure for Advocate at that time.

The senior executive management team at Advocate comprises the CEO and his eight direct reports. Like the streamlined governance

Figure 6.6. Leadership Structure, Advocate Health Care.

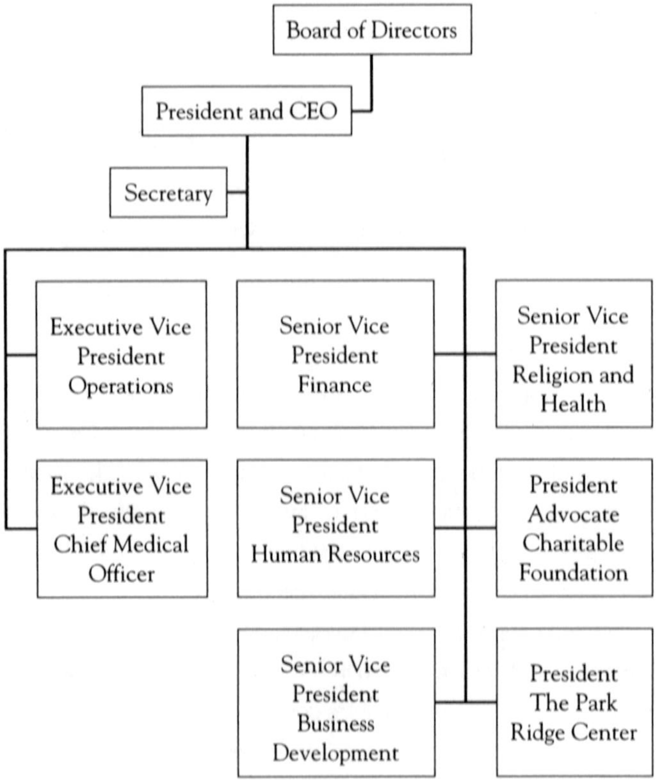

model, this relatively small, focused group of executive leadership has greatly enhanced Advocate's ability to make decisions quickly and facilitate integration throughout the organization. Operating unit management is comparable to that of many of the other systems in this study. Each operating unit has a chief executive responsible for the performance of that specific unit. All hospital operating unit chief executives report directly to the system chief operating officer/executive vice president of operations, and the chief executives for the medical groups report directly to Advocate's chief medical officer. Within each operating unit, leaders of nonclinical support functions (such as human resources, finance, and planning) report through a matrix structure to both the head of the individual operating unit and the head of the functional department at the corporate office. Those who are involved in clinical services have more localized reporting structures confined within each site. To facilitate coordination among the operating units and functions within the operating units, periodic meetings are held with "cross-system" constituents. For example, the chief executives of all the operating units meet monthly to address appropriate systemwide issues.

One key challenge facing Advocate management was concern among operating units regarding consistency and fairness in internal financial reporting and transfer pricing. This proved to be a large barrier, especially in the light of decreasing reimbursement resulting from implementation of the Balanced Budget Act and increased managed care competition in the market. Site management is held responsible for reaching budgets, and there is considerable pressure to meet financial goals. Management is continually evaluating processes and structures that will equitably allocate costs to operating units for services deemed critical for internal corporate development.

Like other systems in the study, incentive compensation proved to be a significant facilitator of management integration at Advocate. The compensation pool reaches a broad group of management based on system overall performance. The overall incentive compensation pool is accrued on a monthly basis. Individual operating unit management compensation is based on achieving key goals in areas including patient and employee satisfaction; financial performance; and mission, vision, and philosophy.

Senior management at Advocate is pleased with the developmental progress and efficiency of the new management structure. There is consensus among management that the integrated system model of delivering health care will be one of the lasting models in the marketplace. Advocate management is getting a head start on developing structures that will facilitate integration of the system. Management is also convinced that its decision to enter into full asset merger affiliations (rather than pursuing more loosely aligned relationships) has had a positive impact on its outcome. Growth through additional mergers, partnerships, or strategic affiliations may be adversely affected, however, by Advocate's preference for full asset merger relationships and the stringent requirements expected of a potential partner.

## Lessons Learned

Senior management realizes that system integration will always be a work in progress and that no organization across the country has a magic bullet that ensures success. It also believes that although the health care market continues to evolve, the integrated system model will survive and become a standard for future organizational structures. In the future, it believes, integrated systems that are tightly managed will outperform those that are loosely organized. Certainly Advocate's strong financial performance, backed by an AA bond rating, coupled with its significant market share gains gives credence to their views.

In addition, management learned that balancing resources among competing priorities takes a significant amount of time and effort to ensure fairness and equity and to maintain harmony among leadership of operating units. Collaborative relationships between operating unit leadership and corporate executive management have been critical to the successful implementation of system strategies.

Advocate management believes that the future of successful health care organizations will be closely linked to their ability to achieve a high degree of system integration. This will include a streamlined decision-making process, an ability to move quickly to take advantage of changes in the market, and better organization around functions critical to achieving the goals of the organization. Management is confident that its new organizational structure will prove to be a key factor in its ability to achieve a high level of system integration. A continued focus on the effectiveness of its governance and management structures and a willingness to make changes where necessary will allow Advocate to achieve its goals and provide value-added services to its customers.

◆　◆　◆　◆　◆　◆

## Fairview Health Services

Fairview Health Services has evolved over the past ninety-four years into a leading regional integrated delivery system. It began with a group of Norwegian Lutherans in Minneapolis who decided that the community needed a hospital to care for those with tuberculosis and a mission that has remained constant over the years: to improve the health of the communities it serves.

Throughout the early and mid-1990s, Fairview entered into multiple merger and affiliation agreements and, as a result, had to make significant accommodations in its governance and management structures. Although these affiliations did not cause Fairview to stray from its original mission, it did challenge senior leadership to develop efficient structures to manage the new and evolving organization. Management realized that the system had grown too large for its management structures and that significant reorganization was necessary. This reorganization was the genesis of the new care system model currently in place at Fairview.

The care system encompasses all care provided to a population by Fairview-owned and -aligned providers, including hospitals, ambulatory care, physician groups, and home care (see Figure 6.7). Fairview defines a care system as "a system of care encompassing the continuum of services (e.g., prevention/primary care specialized, acute inpatient services, end-of-life care) aimed at satisfying community and market need. Community means geographic area,

Figure 6.7. Care System, Fairview Health Services.

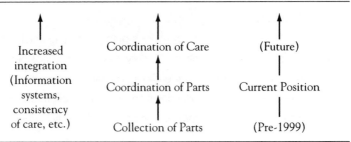

disease-based population segment, market segment, or a group with a common healthcare need" (Fairview Strategic Plan, 1999–2004). Fairview organized its structure around eight care systems: seven geographic areas and one market segment (seniors). Fairview management believes that the care system model will be a critical factor in the organization's future success and its ability to integrate care across the continuum and across the organization.

## Governance

In 1998, Fairview's board assigned a task force to assess its governance function and outline a strategy for the future of governance in the organization (see Figure 6.8). Two key drivers of the assessment were to reduce the number of levels of decision making in the organization and to find an amicable solution to the evolving governance structure necessitated by the mergers and acquisitions of the past decade. The task force found that Fairview's corporate board had grown too large and that there was not a clearly defined role for the local-level governance in the organization.

Today's Fairview's corporate board consists of thirty-seven members. Twenty-four are elected by Fairview's hospitals and other affiliated organizations, seven are elected by the twenty-four elected members as at-large members, and six serve as ex officio members. The ex officio members consist of Fairview's CEO and COO, the chair of the Fairview Foundation, and three University of Minnesota officials. The elected and at-large members are community members and physicians. To streamline the governance function, Fairview's board delegated specific operating authority to its fourteen-member executive committee. The role of the corporate board was redefined to include an educational focus and broader policy-setting and strategic roles.

The relative roles and responsibilities of the operating unit boards were also reviewed and clarified. Typically they have responsibility for local area policy, budgeting, credentialing, human resource decisions, as well as autonomy for capital decision making when projected expenditures are less than $1 million. This provides flexibility in governing

Figure 6.8. Board Structure, Fairview Health Services.

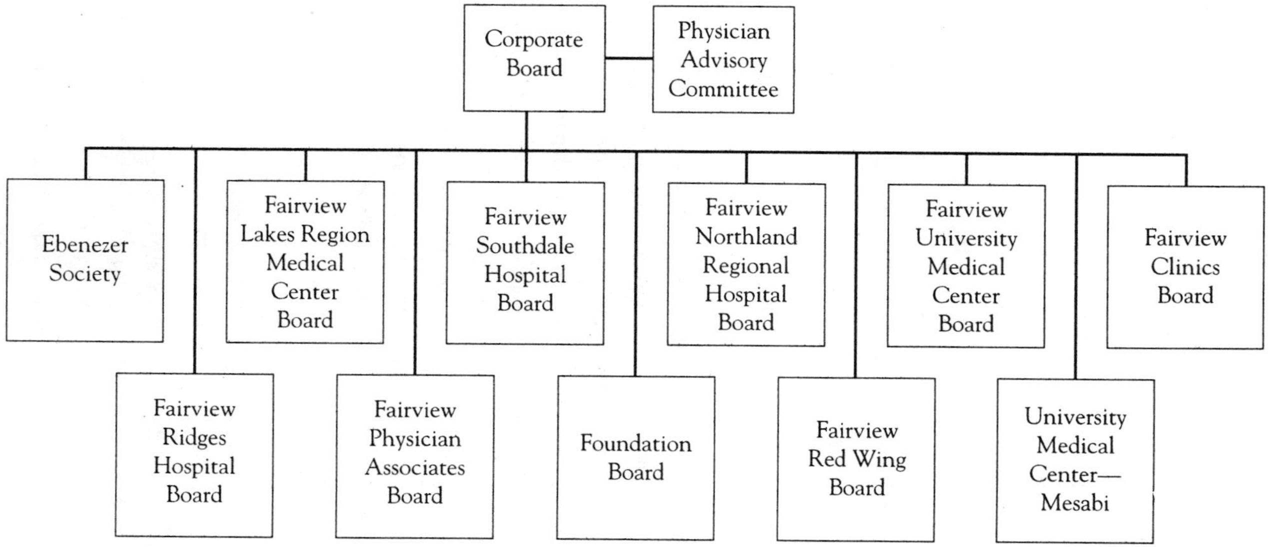

individual operations while simultaneously eliminating unnecessary items from the system board's agenda.

Care system boards exist in some but not all of the care systems in an effort to enhance integration. Currently several of these boards (particularly in greater Minnesota regions) function as governance for entire care systems and spend a large part of their time in decisions for the care system. As care system governance evolves through joint care system boards, activities, strategic, and policy-setting initiatives will become more prevalent on the agenda. These boards are more developed in rural areas than in urban areas, but management believes that this development will occur over time as the system continues to align its economic, business, and organizational models rationally.

The rationale behind the new governance structure was clear: clarify the role and responsibility of the executive committee of the board, eliminate hurdles to accomplishing its mission, and simplify the decision-making process by reducing the number of levels required to make decisions for the organization. Fairview management recognized the importance of its relationship with its governing board members and its communities, and worked diligently to ensure that although board structure and accountability had changed, community input into Fairview governance remained strong.

The new governance structure provides each operating unit the benefit of increased flexibility to achieve its targets. Senior leadership reports that the system of decentralized governance responsibility works very well when operating units are meeting targets, although it does not yet have enough experience to judge how well this arrangement will work when targets are not being met.

A challenge for Fairview's governance will be balancing its ability to decentralize decision making and planning to the care system and operating unit level, while functioning as an integrated whole. Over time, conflicts between operating units, care systems, and the parent organization will likely manifest. Although management reports that this has not been a big issue to date, governing the organization remains an area of constant focus. Management believes that integration will come by energizing local representatives to become more accountable for performance and strategically allocating scarce capital resources.

Through the 1990s, Fairview grew significantly. Its many mergers and acquisitions enabled it to accumulate additional components of the continuum and to broaden its geographic reach as an integrated system. As a result, growing demands are being placed on the trustees of the organization. In the future, diversity of professional experience will play a key role in selecting new board members. Fairview executives will be looking to trustees to provide senior management with a greater level of community understanding, expertise, and perspective, as well as strategies to help the organization have a more heightened consumer focus. To enhance the value that trustees add to the system, management will need to implement a systemwide trustee education and integration forum. This will help board members to understand better the system goals and strategic direction, which enables them to fulfill their role as a trustee.

## Management

Currently, Fairview's formal organizational chart is organized along traditional functional lines (see Figure 6.9). However, as with governance, management at Fairview is evolving to reflect more directly its commitment to the care system model of organization. Each care system has designated a single senior-level executive to lead its efforts. However, depending on the care system, some of these leaders have true managerial accountability for the performance of all the components that define that care system, while others serve more as coordinators of the parts. Care system management meets either monthly or quarterly, depending on its stage of development, to address the needs of the care system and plan additional integration strategies. All care system leadership, with the exception of Fairview Physician Associates and the Fairview University Medical Center (due to its unique partnership with the University Academic Health Center)

Figure 6.9. Management Organization Chart, Fairview Health Services.

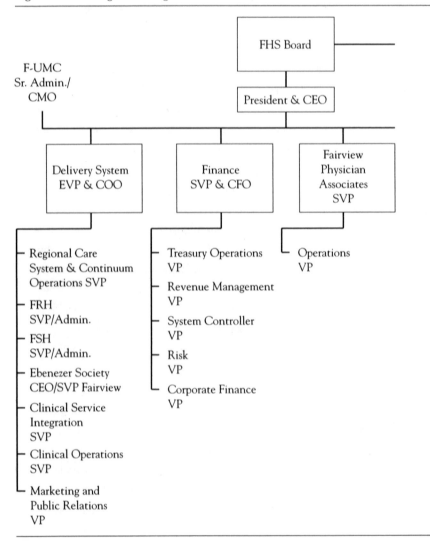

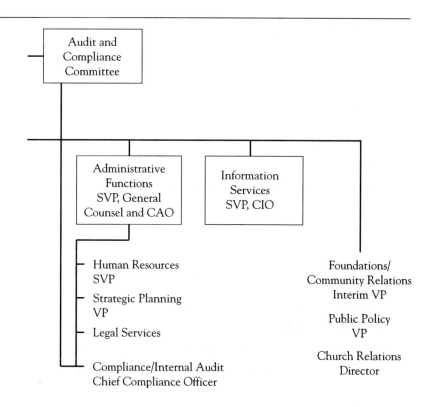

report to the executive vice president (EVP) and chief operating offi-cer (COO). The alignment of reporting adds significantly to the inte-gration of efforts across care systems.

Senior leadership at Fairview functions in a matrix relationship whereby senior vice presidents have both an operating unit–level ac-countability and a system responsibility. Fairview has centralized much of its corporate management functions in an effort to improve coordination and integration of services. Many functions—finance, accounting, strategic development, information systems, human re-sources, and marketing—rely on centralized leadership and staff with support from local functional leaders at individual operating units. As a result of the focus on care systems and the new layer of manage-ment accompanying them, corporate staffs for functions assumed by care systems have been reduced accordingly. Senior leadership has encouraged pushing as much responsibility and staff down to the care system level as possible in an effort to focus management on is-sues at the operating unit level.

To facilitate further functional integration across its system, stream-line management, and reduce overhead costs, Fairview created a number of functional integration teams (FITs) that focus on functions that cut across the system but can be centrally managed to enhance patient satisfaction and quality of care while simultaneously reducing costs. Teams have been created in the following areas:

- Imaging services

- Laboratory services

- Rehabilitation services

- Nutrition services

- Medication management

- Nursing

- Health information management services

- Materials

- Occupancy services

- Emergency services

- Perioperative services

Teams are also being developed for care management and sales. Membership on these teams varies widely, depending on the function under examination. However, typical membership includes department head–level management, as well as front-line employees from multiple areas and operating units. Management reports that over the past two years, over $10 million of annual costs have been eliminated from the system as a result of the work of the functional integration teams. These teams have an administrative director to oversee their day-to-day operations and a senior-level corporate sponsor to assist in eliminating corporate barriers and cross-system issues.

Management reports that its matrix system, coupled with care system development, has significantly improved integration efforts across the system. An excellent example is the systemwide capital allocation process. Fiscal year 1999 marked the first year that capital was allocated by the care systems, then to the individual operating units within the care systems. Care systems had to evaluate the relative necessity of capital requests in terms of value added to the care system's overall strategy and potential contribution to system growth. This process significantly improved the integration of units within care systems. Focus changed from a facility-centric view to a broader vision of understanding the core business and allocating capital accordingly. In the future, this process will be enhanced by a business portfolio analysis that is currently under development. This process will assign business units to one of four categories—cash business, core business, continuum business, or complementary business—and match this with different scenarios in an effort to define strategy for the future. Fairview management expects this model to be operational for the capital allocation process for 2000–2001.

In addition, incentive compensation has played an increasingly important role in focusing management attention on integration efforts. Previously all management incentive compensation was based on overall system performance. Recently the basis for rewarding incentive pay has changed to a model focusing more on individual operating unit performance. Seventy-five percent of incentive compensation is now based on operating unit performance and only 25 percent on overall system performance. As the system continues to evolve and care systems assume responsibility for their overall profitability, this model will change to enhance alignment of incentives. Management is developing a performance measurement tool that will be instrumental in improving future iterations of the incentive compensation model.

One of the key barriers to achieving management integration is the number of merger and acquisition relationships that Fairview management has entered into over the past decade. Focus on completing these mergers has kept management from addressing the hard work of integrating management across operating units and care systems and throughout the organization. In addition, the challenge of updating and modifying systems, facilities, and equipment to be Y2K compliant diverted funds and management attention away from integration activities.

- Fairview management found that an additional challenge in integrating its management structures is maintaining a level focus on other key satisfaction indicators. Although a significant amount of energy and attention is focused internally on developing and integrating the organization, patient and employee satisfaction cannot be ignored. Management must find the right balance between its continued pursuit of integration, while also recommitting its efforts and resources to enhancing the patient and employee experience.

## Lessons Learned

Like other systems across the country, Fairview has had to adjust its management structures in response to the financial pressures resulting from the implementation of the federal Balanced Budget Act.

Management reports that it has eliminated over $10 million of annual costs attributable to corporate overhead. Layers of management were eliminated and positions were realigned, particularly in the urban regions, in an effort to streamline corporate functions. Levels of accountability for financial performance have been increased as each site executive has taken on a heightened responsibility for the site's profitability. Currently, most care system leadership is not responsible for care system profit and loss. Management anticipates that as integration strategies continue to unfold, overall accountability for care system profitability will be evaluated and realigned.

Fairview senior management is convinced that continuing its integration strategy will be imperative for it to be successful in the future. The system has been evolving and growing in order to accumulate all of the pieces necessary to become an integrated delivery system; however, management believes that it has yet to begin to truly add value to the patient experience or deliver value to health care consumers as a result of having all the pieces under one corporate structure. Management is in the beginning stages of a long process designed to integrate governance and management structures across all parts of the health system. Flexibility will be a key ingredient in achieving the next level of management integration. Different organizational structures may be required to maximize the success of its efforts; however, execution of integration strategies will be the key determinant for Fairview to realize the full benefits of becoming a truly integrated delivery system.

## Sentara Healthcare

Sentara Healthcare (Sentara), like many of the study systems, has grown over the years to join the ranks of the nation's large, comprehensive, regional health systems. Having opened its doors as the Retreat for the Sick in 1888, Sentara has continued to focus on serving the health care needs of eastern Virginia and northeastern North Carolina for more than one hundred years.

In the past few years, Sentara has formed several joint-venture relationships. In June 1998, it merged operations with Tidewater Health Care (Tidewater) to broaden the system's reach and strengthen its not-for-profit mission in the region. This significant change prompted management to reassess its system strategic plan to ensure that the new structure and the existing plan were congruent. Strategically, Sentara recommitted itself to a focus on the consumer through:

- Development of the clinically excellent operating model
- Enhancing knowledge of consumer needs to create value-driven products and services
- Evolving physician alliances, both strategic and financial
- Enhancing Sentara Health Management (an owned insurance company) capabilities and expanding financing options
- Building access, knowledge, and connectivity capabilities, including retail business and Internet strategies

Strategies during the past twenty years focused on building the integrated delivery system, developing it regionally, and increasing the number of covered lives in the health plans. This new strategic direction reflects a distinct shift in focus from the strategies of the past. The new Sentara strategic plan seeks to improve health care by responding to consumer-defined optimal health care experiences and providing demonstrably optimal outcomes.

## Governance

Sentara's governance structure is the most consolidated of any of the systems studied. The current board meets ten times each year and comprises twenty-six members. Twenty percent of the board membership is made up of physicians. Sentara management noted that its corporate charter does not require a specific physician class of board membership. Physicians are elected to the board as members of the community, not to specifically represent its physician constituency.

Over the next three years, the new board will be streamlined to fourteen individuals. The evolution of a leaner governance structure is an intentional effort to consolidate decision making and facilitate implementation. Sentara CEO David Bernd noted that although the decision to reduce the size of the board was difficult, it was agreed to by the merger partners and incorporated in the merger documents. An additional factor in the smooth merger transition was significant input and strong leadership from the chairman of Sentara's board. These factors have helped to minimize the emotional barriers and political struggles often associated with reducing board size and membership.

Sentara highlights its lean governance structure as one of its strongest assets. The board of directors holds all accountability and responsibility for governing the health system. Additional subsidiary boards exist only as regulatory requirements dictate. These include Sentara Health Management, medical group boards, and Williamsburg Community Hospital (a joint venture). Each of these boards functions subordinately to the Sentara corporate board and does not have any fiduciary responsibility. There are no subsidiary boards at the hospital level.

Sentara's corporate board functions with four standing committees (medical affairs, finance, audit, and compensation); committee membership is predominantly board members. All board work that does not fit within the auspices of these four committees is delegated to task forces. Sentara President Douglas Johnson noted that the advantage of task forces is that they can focus on a specific issue and then, once the issue has been resolved, disband. Too often, standing committees outlive their usefulness and simply waste people's time. CEO Bernd also noted that this heavy emphasis on task forces gives the organization a huge advantage by creating a very effective and efficient method of governing.

In the 1980s, Sentara's governance structure functioned in a more decentralized manner. Boards were established for each hospital as well as specific services (such as geriatrics, ambulatory care, etc.). In the early 1990s, Sentara made the decision to consolidate these boards into one system board in order to maintain focus on system goals. Management is pleased with the new centralized structure and is convinced that this is one of the reasons the merger transition has gone so smoothly and the organization is functioning so well.

## Management

The executive-level decision making is consolidated into a group of six senior managers: the CEO, president, EVP–COO care delivery, SVP chief medical officer, SVP finance, and SVP managed care (see Figure 6.10). This group, called the Committee of the CEO, is responsible for establishing goals, assigning agendas, monitoring progress, developing external policy, "tie-breaking," developing financial strategy, approving budgets, allocating strategic capital, and assigning interdivisional projects.

To supplement traditional lines of reporting and facilitate cross-system coordination, a systemwide committee structure (see Figure 6.11) was created to address three critically strategic areas of focus for the organization. Each committee has clearly defined functions and reports to the Committee of the CEO, with final decisions made by the CEO. Sentara's president chairs the Strategy, Analysis, and Support Committee, which is charged with developing corporate strategy, implementing and monitoring the strategy, recommending allocation of strategic capital, and developing new business opportunities. The chief medical officer chairs the Medical Management Committee. This committee is responsible for all medical management across Sentara, physician relationship building, physician integration, clinical quality, and clinical effectiveness. The Operations Management Committee is chaired by the chief operating officer and is accountable for financial performance review, operations review, and decisions regarding operating capital allocation.

Many functional areas at Sentara, such as strategic planning, work in a top-down, bottom-up fashion. Overall strategic direction for the organization is the responsibility of the Committee of the CEO, with responsibility for implementation delegated to the Strategy,

Analysis, and Support Committee. Once the strategic planning process is complete at the system level, individual operating units are responsible for developing site-level strategies. These strategies must fit within the strategic direction outlined by the system strategic plan. This structure allows for centralization of strategy development for different functions, and it requires individual operating units to fit site-level strategies within the framework developed by the system. Management believes that strategic decision making will be crucial to its success in the future.

Sentara management believes that involving physicians in key leadership positions is vital to its success. Eighteen physicians are currently in full-time or part-time senior management positions throughout the system. The Medical Management Committee has also established two physician committees comprising twelve practicing physicians, one committee for each of Sentara's distinct markets.

The decision to develop this new management structure was driven by the need to focus management's attention on internal integration. Combining two different cultures, operations, management staffs, etc., requires a tight senior management structure and a consistent message from the top of the organization. A commitment to integrate the three key operational components of the system (facilities, health plans, and physicians) has been essential.

In addition to these groups of senior leadership in the organization, a "Reinventing Sentara" team has been working on specific management challenges for the last five years. This group is made up of middle managers and executives; it functions like a think tank, focusing on issues critical to improving overall practices within the system. Senior management believes that this group is of such importance that members are eligible to take a leave of absence for as long as two years from their current positions to participate. The commitment to Reinventing Sentara is firm, although the group has experienced both successes and failures. Among some of its more notable successes are an improved process to manage costs and a realigned patient care approach, which includes systemwide case

Figure 6.10. Sentara Healthcare Corporate Officers.

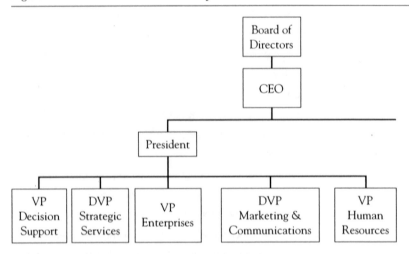

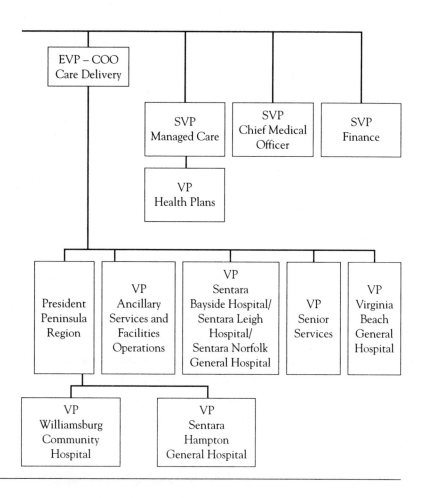

Figure 6.11. Sentara Healthcare Committee Structure.

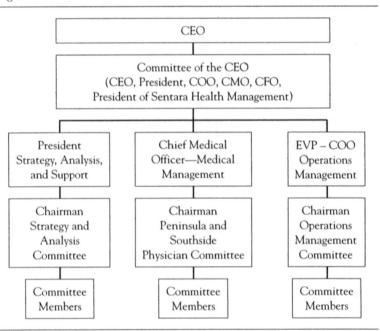

management. Management is constantly developing strategies to enhance the success of the group. Encouraging departments and divisions to come to Reinventing Sentara with ideas for improvements in costs and quality rather than forcing change on departments has enhanced implementation. Managers and teams that successfully implement cost or quality enhancements can win awards for doing so (for instance, the CEO Award). Overall, management believes that Reinventing Sentara has served its purpose well.

## Lessons Learned

Key lessons were learned as a result of the merger and the reevaluation of the governance and management structures. Although it may sound simplistic, management believes that one of the keys to its ability to integrate its organization and make it successful was a focus on the basics. CEO Bernd acknowledged that working on the basics is not very glamorous, but he indicated that many people avoid it because foundation building is time consuming and difficult. He believes that not doing so is a big mistake because there is a great payback to building a solid foundation. Additionally, Sentara senior management had to eliminate the subsidy mentality. Bernd noted that "cross-subsidization is the death knell of integrated health care." A premise in the Sentara organization is that every subsidiary has to make it on its own, and that each has to have a positive bottom line. Management is constantly evaluating the organization and eliminating cross-subsidization wherever possible.

Channeling decisions down to the appropriate decision makers and providing decisions in a timely way has called for flexibility and good communication. Additionally, communicating across an organization of twelve thousand people, among them eight hundred managers at one level or another, presents management with an added degree of complexity. As a condition of approving the Sentara-Tidewater merger, federal regulators required an economic impact study to be completed. A component of the merger requirements was a commitment from management to generate cost savings in excess of $50 million from the combined organization over the first five years. Management reports that it is well on the way to achieving this goal. In order to facilitate integration of processes, systems, and people, teams were formed to identify and implement cost savings cited in the economic impact study. (Savings must maintain or improve quality and processes.) Management's philosophy has been to draw from the best of both, or seek out a new best practice.

A key determinant to the success of this effort is overall FTE management. To date, consolidations of like departments and divisions have had smooth transitions thanks to attrition and opportunities within the organization. Management is committed to achieving (and exceeding) the $50 million savings goal.

Sentara management articulated several best practices that have enabled the organization to succeed in becoming more tightly integrated. Internal communication played a key role not only in keeping the organization informed but also in beginning to develop a new corporate culture. Many communication methods were employed, both formal and informal. In addition, a systemwide management meeting is held every six months to reexamine and update, at a high level, the integration efforts and successes and failures. Management also periodically reexamines the overall structure of the system and its effectiveness. In countless institutions, it is too often the case that systems are organized by informal means and left that way. Although examining the organization and making changes has emotional and political implications, regular analysis helps the organization evolve to meet its current needs and prevents significant deviations from the agreed-upon structure.

As noted in other case studies, incentive programs have played a key role in developing organizations' integration efforts and overall success. Sentara Healthcare uses both short-term and long-term programs with separate goals for specific clinical quality and financial success for senior management. For the rank and file, there is a gain-sharing program called Resultshare, which is both innovative and inclusive. All employees in the organization (except senior executives) are eligible to receive an annual bonus payment based on several factors. The key driving variables are financial performance and customer satisfaction. Both goals are imperative to Sentara's success and are measured in the program.

In order for Resultshare to be funded, a 2 percent operating margin must be achieved before benefits can be awarded. Once this threshold has been reached, customer satisfaction goals must be met. Management reports that the largest impact of this program has been improved customer satisfaction. The program is based equally on system and divisional results. Two positive outcomes of the program are that (1) employees consider not only department or division goals but also systemwide goals and (2) employees across the organization are much more aware of financial performance. A large portion of senior management pay is determined by a separate long-term incentive program. Bernd noted that gainsharing for employees is used throughout the organization because of the upside potential for gain and absence of downside risk, whereas the senior management program has both upside potential and downside risk.

Management has made significant strides in the last five years to develop Sentara Healthcare into one of the leading integrated delivery systems in the country. This has occurred both in spite of and as a result of its affiliation activities. Management realizes that the changes it has made in the last few years are part of a long-term iterative process of developing management and governance uniquely structured to meet the health care needs of the communities it serves. By remaining flexible and willing to change, and ensuring that structures do not get in the way of producing results, Sentara management has positioned the organization to maximize the benefits of becoming an integrated delivery system.

# Integrated Health Care and the Community Health Care Management System

## Prospects for the Future

Implementing the promise of integrated health care will continue to be slow and uneven. The momentum for integration created by the prospects of national health care reform in 1994 has been slowed. Capitated payment placing providers at risk has not evolved across the country to the extent predicted. Integration efforts have been largely limited to "size wars" involving financial and legal transactions designed to achieve greater market presence in order to negotiate more favorable rates with health plans. As a result, very little true management of patient care or creation of value has occurred. Almost everyone is playing around the edges with the hope that the game can be won across the merger table or the contract negotiation table without entering the physician's clinic, the patient's home, or getting involved in community health issues. No one is yet serious enough about value improvement, never mind continuous value improvement. No one is yet willing to invest in value improvement because they are unsure that it will be recognized by the marketplace or governmental purchasers of care. Few are willing to take the first steps.

Given this situation, most systems are on the precipice of having stranded their integration building assets and capabilities in the sense of not yet being able to convert them to value for purchasers. For some, this is because they have had difficulty moving beyond assembling the pieces of integration. For other systems, it is because they continue to operate largely in functional silos. For still others, it is because they have had understandable problems in developing effective partnerships with physicians, many of whom exhibit an "under siege" mentality. Everyone recognizes that the task of achieving clinical integration depends on so many variables that one hardly knows where to begin.

And that is not all. The energy, focus, and financial resources needed to address these challenges have been severely eroded by a confluence of events that have left most systems' economic moorings shaky. These include the negative financial impact of the Balanced Budget Act of 1997, the ratcheting down of payment rates by Medicare and Medicaid HMOs, the steep rise in pharmaceutical costs, and the need to reengineer computer systems to deal with Y2K compliance. Any one of these alone would have posed financial challenges; all four coming together has resulted in severe financial losses for many study systems—for some, the first in their history. Investment income from a strong economy has temporarily saved the day. But it is difficult for physicians to work with diabetic patients on insulin control when the physician's very practice is threatened. It is difficult to implement practice guidelines and diffuse them to other operating units throughout the system when the staff for doing so has been cut by 50 percent. It is not possible to make progress with clinical integration initiatives when, due to financial losses, you've had to "kill it off." In the descriptive words of one study respondent, "Clinical integration is fine when things are going well and you can focus on it. But it's difficult to do when you have a gun held to your head." We would add that integration is not something that can be simply turned on and off, depending on the vicissitudes of the environment.

This is not a picture that is being presented. It is a reality that is being lived. So why are these systems persisting in their commitment to integrated health care delivery? We think there are three answers, and the study systems reflect two of these three. First, for some it is a matter of principle, mission, and vision. These systems believe it is the best way to deliver health care. They are in it for the long run, regardless of the obstacles in their path. We might call them the "true believers." The second group is not really sure which direction health care is going to go in the future and thus view integration as an adaptation strategy. These systems want to be prepared to move in whatever direction the wind blows, and they see the "integration journey" as a process that will help them build experience and capabilities to switch strategies as the environment demands (for example, from ownership to contractual relationships or vice versa). Thus, they want some experience with centralization as well as decentralization, with standardization and flexibility, with multiple relationships with physicians, and so on (Institute for Health and Aging, 1996). We might call these systems the "fence sitters." They believe (or hope) that an integrating strategy will give them a higher perch on the fence from which they can get a better look at what might be coming down the road and a little more time to prepare.

The third group, not represented by any of our study systems but found outside the study sample, is not sure at all about the benefits of integration but also does not see viable alternatives. Integration still seems to make sense to these systems on paper and it "sounds right" to them. This group desperately wants to believe in it and see it work. We might call this group the "faith seekers."

Whether a true believer, a fence sitter, or a faith seeker, systems have modified their approach to integrated health care delivery over the past four years. Among the most prevalent developments have been these:

- A growing recognition that health care delivery value is created locally and a resulting movement toward greater decentralization and sharing of functional support services with local regions and within local regions with local delivery units

- The growth of blended models of centralization and decentralization, whereby greater operational control is granted to individual operating units while overall strategic control and direction are maintained by the system

- A greater emphasis on basic principles, or what we have called "robust factors," that underlie effective physician partnerships as opposed to preoccupation with specific organizational models

- An increased appreciation for the difficulty of achieving clinical integration and therefore a movement toward greater focus by working on specific pieces of it

- Greater attention given to mixing vertical integration ownership models with virtual integration contractual, strategic alliance, and outsourcing approaches

But these adaptive changes are not likely to result in a marked breakthrough of progress in integrated health care delivery over the next few years. The negative forces—lack of aligned economic incentives, lack of a coherent national health policy, lack of a business case for quality or value, and continuing pressures on financial bottom lines—are simply too strong. Instead, we foresee a ten- to fifteen-year time horizon that will, in an evolutionary fashion, result in more integrated health care delivery as part of a larger community health care management system, a concept introduced in our original book. We believe five interrelated forces will push U.S. health care in this direction over approximately the next fifteen years (see Table 7.1).

## Five Forces and Fifteen Years

The five forces are an aging population, technology, the empowered consumer, payment innovations, and the ability to partner.

Table 7.1. Integration Building Blocks over Time.

| | |
|---|---|
| 1995–Present ➤ | Age of Functional Integration[a] |
| 2000–2005 ➤ | Age of Physician Integration[b] |
| 2006–2010 ➤ | Age of Clinical Integration[c] |
| 2010–2015 ➤ | Age of Population-Based Health Management[d] |

[a]Human resources, financial management, marketing, strategic planning, information management, and TQM brought together to focus on patient needs across the continuum of care.

[b]Sustainable trusting relationships developed between physician organizations and other entities to facilitate the redesign of patient care.

[c]The right services provided in the right time and place and coordinated across time, place, and providers to meet patient needs. The seamless continuum of care is a reality.

[d]The goals and actions of the health care system are driven by the prioritized health needs of the community. The health delivery system works with other community health—building assets to maintain, restore, and enhance the health of individuals and the community at large. Primary emphasis is placed on prevention, early intervention, and health promotion. Providers are paid based on health outcomes achieved.

## Aging

One-third of the population will reach age sixty-five in the year 2011; by 2030, 21.5 percent of the population will be over age sixty-five. Many of these individuals will have chronic illness of multiple forms that will become increasingly severe with advancing age. Nearly 90 percent of people over age sixty-five have at least one chronic condition, and 70 percent of those have more than one (Institute for Health and Aging, 1996). The most prevalent chronic conditions are arthritis, hypertension, heart disease, sensory and mobility impairments, diabetes, and dementia. Their needs are not likely to be effectively met by isolated focused factories or narrowly organized microsystems. Care coordination capabilities will be needed of a sort that many organized delivery systems are trying to build into their integrated health care models today. But traditional managed care models do not really engage in care management of the very sick. As others have noted, it could well be the Achilles' heel of managed care (Anders, 1996; Kleinke, 1998). In brief, as the population continues to age and the number of individuals with multiple chronic illness grows, we foresee a great demand for more integrated models of care that can truly work with the elderly and their adult children in coordinating across multiple providers and sites over time. It will also involve considerable interface with the mental health, social services, assisted living, and other sectors of the community given the increased need of many elderly for these services.

### Technology

A second major driving force toward the development of more integrated health care delivery in a population-based health model will be the acceleration of developments in the biomedical sciences, biotechnology, pharmaceuticals, and information technology—what we call the "bio-med, bio-tech, pharma-tech, and info-tech" revolution. As the results of the Human Genome Project are implemented in clinical practice, it becomes possible to foresee and predict the health needs of individuals and groups over their life span. Further, through genetic and related forms of "engineering," it becomes possible to intervene to correct or improve the health problems identified. Although it is possible to argue that these developments may lead to still greater specialization and growth of focused factories (for example, for spina bifida, Parkinson's disease, breast cancer, or Alzheimer's disease), we believe the actual care interventions implied by the new technologies will require coordination across multiple providers and experts and also heavy mental, social, emotional, and spiritual components of care.

Information technology will play a special role in providing more integrated health care delivery in two major ways. First, it gives consumers a powerful tool for helping to manage and integrate their own care in partnership with physicians, nurses, and other members of the health professional team. Second, it extends the integrative capability of physicians, nurses, and health professionals and care systems at large through the ability to manage patients from a distance through Internet, call center, and telemed line technologies. Call centers are already moving from being used primarily as marketing, referral, and scheduling functions to more sophisticated disease and demand management of patients with both acute and chronic illness (Coile, 1999; Barr, Laufenberg, and Sieckman, 1998).

### The Empowered Consumer

The combination of the first two forces—aging and technology—will provide the fuel for the age of the empowered consumer. The baby boomer generation will be the driving force behind both greater choice in health care delivery and greater use of electronic information technology to help inform those choices. Combined with the availability of new treatments to both extend and improve the quality of life, we can expect a growing consumer voice in all aspects of health care delivery. The empowerment will take place at both an individual and a collective level. At the individual level, consumers will have greater on-line access to clinical information (Coile, 1999). There are more than twenty-five thousand health-related Web sites available (Berwick, 1998), and it is estimated that about half of the American population will have access to the Internet at home (Mittman and Cain, 1999). Even though illness will still place consumers in a position of vulnerability, increased access to the information will provide a healthier balance and foster greater mutual discussion among patients, their physicians, and the health care team at large. Physicians and other members of the team will serve more as coaches and co-managers, with patients as guardians and promoters of the patients' health. Patients will become actively involved in self-management of chronic illnesses such as heart disease, asthma, diabetes, and depression (Center for the Advancement of Health, 1999). If recent trends continue, it is likely that the health care team will also be expanded to include chiropractors, massage therapists, and other providers of complementary medicine. For example, between 1990 and 1997, there was an increase from 34 percent to 42 percent in the percentage of Americans using alternative therapies and a 63 percent increase in the total volume of visits, from 386 million to 629 million, exceeding the 427 million visits made to all primary care physicians in 1997 (Eisenberg and others, 1998).

On a collective basis, consumers organized as employer purchaser coalitions are likely to push for increased accountability for costs and we believe, over time, for quality and outcomes of care as well. The business health care action group (BHCAG) in the Twin Cities of Minnesota, the Pacific Business Group on Health in California, and the Missouri Department of Health (see Tables 7. 2 and 7.3) among others are now routinely providing data on various quality indicators by plans, hospitals, and, in some cases, individual physician groups. The goal is to provide accurate, relevant data to corporate purchasers on the theory that they will purchase on "value criteria" related to the combination of cost, quality, and outcomes of care that best meet their needs and preferences. The Pacific Business Group on Health has taken this reporting to a new level by prospectively negotiating performance guarantees with thirteen of California's largest HMOs (Schauffler, Brown, and Milstein, 1999). If the targets are not met, money is refunded by the HMOs to the Pacific Business Group on Health. The evidence that such collective reporting and public accountability will change employer consumer behavior is somewhat mixed. For example, after ten years, the Cleveland Health Quality Choice Program organized by Cleveland's major employers was dissolved despite indications that death rates fell significantly after Health Quality Choice begin publishing its reports (Sirio and Harper, 1996). For the most part, employers simply did not shift patients to the better-performing hospitals, particularly after the rapid rise in costs in the mid-1990s begin to subside (Burton, 1999). However, we believe that major pressure in the future for value purchasing will come from the Medicare and Medicaid programs in addition

Table 7.2.  Quality Indicators for Medicare Managed Care Plans.

| | Breast Cancer Screening Rate | Diabetic Eye Exam Rate | Mental Health Hospitalization Follow-up Rate | Mental Health Readmission Rate |
|---|---|---|---|---|
| Advantra | High | High | Average | Average |
| BlueCHOICE Senior | Average | Average | Not applicable | Not applicable |
| United HealthCare Medicare Complete | Low | Low | Low | High |
| Statewide managed care average | 68% | 42% | 50% | 21% |
| National managed care average[a] | 71% | 39% | Unknown | Unknown |

| | Doctors Who Communicate Well | Getting Referrals to Specialists | Overall Rating of Care Received | Overall Plan Rating |
|---|---|---|---|---|
| Advantra | Low | Average | Average | High |
| BlueCHOICE Senior | High | Average | Average | Average |
| United HealthCare Medicare Complete | Average | Low | Average | High |
| Statewide managed care average | 72% | 92% | 48% | 51% |

[a]Based on data submitted to the National Committee for Quality Assurance (NCQA). Not all managed care plans do so.

Source: Missouri Department of Health (1998).

Table 7.3. Quality Indicators for Medicaid Managed Care Plans.

| | Rate of Prenatal Care in First Trimester | Cesarean Section Rate | Vaginal Birth After Cesarean Rate | Cervical Cancer Screen Rate | Childhood Immunization Rate |
|---|---|---|---|---|---|
| CARE PARTNERS | Average | Average | Average | High | Low |
| Community Care Plus | Low | High | Average | No report of data | No report of data |
| Healthcare USA of Missouri | Average | Low | Low | Low | Low |
| Mercy MC+ | Average | Average | Average | High | No report of data |
| Prudential HealthCare Community Plan | Average | Average | Average | Average | Low |
| Statewide managed care average | 68% | 16% | 36% | 33% | 7% |
| Statewide non–managed care average | 74% | 21% | 28% | Unknown | Unknown |
| National goal | 90% | 15% | None | 85% | 90% |

| | Checkup Wait 7 Days or Fewer | Minor Injury Rate 3 Days or Fewer | Wait in Office Less Than 1 Hour | Treated Politely | Enough Doctors | Plan Recommendation |
|---|---|---|---|---|---|---|
| CARE PARTNERS | Average | Average | Average | Average | Average | Low |
| Community Care Plus | Low | Average | Average | Average | Average | No report of data |
| Healthcare USA of Missouri | Average | Average | Average | High | Average | Low |
| Mercy MC+ | High | Average | Average | High | High | No report of data |
| Prudential HealthCare Community Plan | Average | Average | Average | Average | Low | Low |
| Statewide managed care average: | 64% | 83% | 83% | 88% | 82% | 7% |

*Source:* Missouri Department of Health (1998).

to the private sector. Together they will provide the impetus for making more data available to both individual consumers and those who purchase on their behalf.

Finally, it is important to note that federal and state efforts associated with patient protection legislation and development of a medical quality review body will reinforce the empowered consumer movement. For example, some have suggested the development of a securities exchange–like commission that would require compulsory registration and public disclosure of costs, utilization, benefits, quality, and outcomes data on a timely basis by health plans and their associated provider groups (Tyson, 1999).

## Payment Innovations

We do not currently pay providers for integrated care. We do not pay providers for the outcomes of care produced. We do not pay for health. It is not likely that this will change quickly. As a result, over the next few years, organized delivery systems and those associated with them will continue to experience financial barriers to creating value through more integrated care experiences.

But there are certain subterranean forces at work that could change payment dynamics by 2005 or so. Perhaps the most important is the growing role played by the public sector through the growth in numbers and expenditures associated with the Medicare and Medicaid programs. As noted by Whitelaw and Warden (1999):

> Medicare reform must support a coordinated health care delivery system (in place of hospital-centered fragmented care) and pro-active chronic disease management (in place of episodic, reactive care). Consumers, government, community-based agencies, employers, health plans, and others need to develop a shared understanding of what outcomes we want to obtain, what delivery system reforms are required, and how financing can support those reforms.

The health care system will be challenged as never before to manage the health of these groups within fixed sums of money. Much of this will involve the management of chronic illness that will push the management of patient care risk to its limits. Most of the risk will continue to be transferred to providers or shared between providers and health plans (including Medicare and Medicaid as payers). Most providers remain behind the curve in their ability to manage risk because they are trying to do it with old mind-sets and practice technologies. Risk cannot be managed on a one-to-one base characterized by the treatment of individual patients alone. It is necessary to take a population-based perspective that enables scarce resources to be used across a population of individuals and provides interventions to keep people well. It also requires providers to rethink how they might interact with the population to manage the risk. For example, the physician or clinic office visit was the core delivery technology of the twentieth century. Is this the best way to deliver health care in the twenty-first century? To what extent will it be replaced or at least complemented by the Internet, group visits, and telemedicine? Most of the previous chapters have discussed the nine systems' progress in expanding their capabilities to truly manage care and patient risk.

But as others have noted (Goldsmith, 1996), managing patient risk is still largely a cost-savings financial management game even if one's focus is on populations and prevention. But what if one were to pay providers based on health outcomes produced (Kindig, 1997, 1998)? Although there are significant technical and political challenges to implementing such a payment scheme, the basic idea is to identify a group of people for whom a given organized delivery system is responsible and determine those aspects of health for which the organized delivery system can exert a reasonable degree of control. Arrangements need to be developed whereby the ODS is not held responsible for individuals who continue to pursue unhealthy behaviors. Payment is then made based on improving the health of the population as measured by health-adjusted life expectancy. This will force health care providers to develop effective linkages with educational, social service, and related community agencies. Models of such collaboration are expanding (Newcomer, Harrington, Friedlob, 1990; Bogue, Antia, Harmata, and Hall, 1997; Kreuter and Lezin, 1998) such that by 2010, it may be possible to develop payment arrangements that provide incentives for health produced.

### Ability to Partner

Although the first four forces are largely external to health care delivery systems, the fifth force—the ability to partner—is largely an internal response. This partnering must occur both within the traditional health sector and across sectors. Health care delivery has become bigger than any one stakeholder can manage: corporate purchaser, federal or state government, health plans, providers, or citizen groups. All must share in the risk, and each must take responsibility and hold each other accountable. The degree and pace of progress with regard to integrated health care delivery will depend on accepting this realization and implementing partnerships that can help achieve mutually shared objectives. Such "collaborative networks" (Mintzberg and Glouberman, 1997) can become the foundation for integrated patient care management, managing patient exposure to health risk, and comprehensive population health care management.

The principles of core competence and comparative advantage are key to building effective partnerships. Core competencies refer to those things that an organization is truly good at doing that are central to its business—that is, to its mission of why the organization exists. Comparative advantage refers to those things that the organization does better than others; they may or may not be considered core to the business or mission, but they can be generally performed better than most others. In the past four years, the study systems have learned more about both their core competencies and comparative advantages from the increased financial pressures and demands for greater accountability. Relationships between and among hospitals, health plans, and physician organizations have been restructured. If anything, ODS leaders are looking for more outsourcing opportunities and strategic partnerships. As Goldsmith (1998a, p. 6) notes, "They must divest, shut down, or take minority ownership interest in the services or businesses they have not mastered; and they must rely upon strategic alliances with suppliers, competitors, health plans, physician practice management firms, and other enterprises to accomplish what they formerly did with in-house resources."

One thing no system should do, however, is to outsource its core competence. The profound realization of most of the study systems over the past four years is that their core competence is indeed the delivery of acute inpatient care. Thus, they own their hospitals. But attempts to develop core competencies in financing and insurance or delivery of comprehensive primary care through ownership of health plans or physician group practices are being severely questioned. Several systems, such as Advocate, Sutter, and Sisters of Providence (Seattle region), have sold their health plans, choosing to redeploy the capital into their core competence of direct care provision. Owned physician groups have been supplemented by loose strategic alliances and contractual relationships (see Chapter Four). And even those that own physician groups are looking for ways to provide greater innovation and entrepreneurial incentives though decentralizing operational activities. In brief, there appears to be a developing trend toward greater virtual integration across levels of care and in relationships among hospitals, health plans, and physician organizations.

A key question must be asked: To what extent are these newly emerging virtual relationships *strategic?* They are strategic only to the extent that the parties involved believe they can achieve their goals and objectives better through partnering with each other than partnering with someone else or going it alone. Thus, it is possible for strategic alliances and partnerships to exist without any common or shared objectives regarding the provision of more integrated patient care. For example, physicians may wish to enter into a PHO arrangement with a hospital for purposes of gaining managed care contracting expertise, while the hospital hopes to gain a greater patient base for admissions and referrals. We refer to these types of strategic alliances as *instrumental* in that they are intended for each partner to achieve its separate objectives.

A second type of strategic alliance exists where two or more partners come together to achieve a *shared* goal or objective that neither can achieve alone. Although these are seldom without "enlightened self-interests," they tend to be more externally focused on achievement of a shared vision. For example, an ODS may partner with a community health organization to reduce teenage pregnancy, substance abuse, or domestic violence. We refer to these partnerships as *symbiotic*.

Both of these forms of alliances are *trading* alliances (Zajac, D'Aunno, and Burns, 2000) in the sense of involving the exchange of different resources and capabilities to create value. They are in contrast to *pooling* alliances in which resources of two or more organizations are simply pooled to benefit all members, without any direct exchange of other assets or capabilities. Health care purchasing alliances serve as a prime example.

It is generally believed that more value can be created through trading alliances in which partners' comparative abilities complement each other, but these alliances are also the most difficult to implement because they involve exchanges of resources that must be coordinated. This involves several challenges. First are the transaction costs of monitoring agreements (Williamson, 1981; Williamson and Ouchi, 1981; Robinson, 1999b). Second is the internal resistance within each partnership that comes from individuals' resenting having to share resources or having their decision making constrained (Annison and Wilford, 1998). Third is the fact that often the organizations involved have different cultures that must be managed. Goldsmith (1998a, p. 7) touches on all of these when he notes, "To tell managers and professionals who have spent their entire lives trying to be organizationally self sufficient, they must now work constructively with outsiders to accomplish their goals is profoundly counter-cultural."

In the next five years or so, hospitals, health plans, physician organizations, and other health care entities will continue their experiments in partnering based on a variety of virtual strategic alliances. But to create real value and an ability to manage risk in a comprehensive fashion, these partnerships will need to expand beyond the health care sector to embrace the community at large.

## The Community Health Care Management System

The goal of the community health care management system is to maintain and enhance the health of individuals, groups, and the community at large, broadly defined to include all components of health: physical, mental, emotional, and spiritual. The medical care system focuses on restoring people with illness, injury, or disease to an improved state of health. The broader health care system, particularly primary care, focuses largely on disease prevention and health maintenance efforts. Both medical care and health care interventions are largely aimed at individuals and thereby are difficult to leverage to improve the overall health status of the community. To accomplish this third objective, it is necessary to link medical care and health care delivery efforts to a broad array of community health-building assets, including educational, family, religious, housing, employment, environmental, legal, and the business sectors. The community health care management system explicitly links the medical care, health care delivery, and community health building assets. As shown in Figure 7.1 the community health-building assets form the platform to help leverage the medical and health care delivery sectors' efforts to restore and maintain health, with all parties working toward enhancing the community's stock of health. The goal is to "push to the left": to push the chronically ill in the community to becoming "sporadically well" and, where possible, "chronically well" and to push the sporadically ill to becoming chronically well.

Figure 7.1. Population-Based Health Continuum Goal:
Creating the Chronically Well.

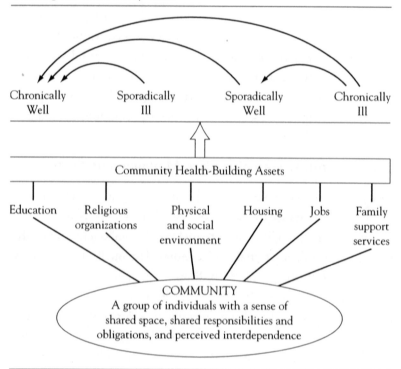

The building blocks of the community health care management
system are shown in Figure 7.2. It begins with obtaining a deep
knowledge of the community's health needs and understanding of
the factors associated with those needs, including the role to be
played by schools and employment, housing, environmental, and
law enforcement agencies. This requires not only creative use of
existing data but also linkage of data from different sources, collection of targeted primary data, and meetings with community residents. The incidence, prevalence, and duration of identified
conditions must be documented. Where possible, the data should
be segmented by age, gender, geographical location, income, insurance status, household size, and related variables. Once these

Figure 7.2.  Building Blocks of the
Community Health Care Management System.

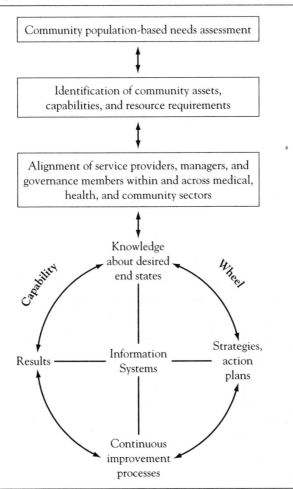

analyses are completed, priorities need to be determined based on both the community's preference and values *and* cost-benefit and cost-effectiveness analysis.

Although identifying and prioritizing the community's health needs is logically prior to determining the configuration of resources to address those needs, these activities can and should be done concurrently. This is shown in the second box of Figure 7.2. The community should assess its strengths, weaknesses, opportunities, and threats (SWOT analysis) associated with its efforts to improve community health. For example, a community may have obvious strengths in a strong base of hospitals and health providers; an untapped strength in a large number of well-educated elderly who can form a pool of potential volunteers; a weakness in the lack of mechanisms to coordinate and leverage the strengths of the provider sector with the educational, social service, and law enforcement sectors of the community; an opportunity afforded by new community leadership and the availability of foundation funding; and, perhaps, a threat posed by conflicting state regulations or diminished federal funding. The SWOT analysis approach goes beyond merely identifying the community's assets or capacity (McKnight, 1995) by taking a more strategic approach to assessing the community's capabilities in relation to the threats and opportunities that it faces. Such an assessment will enable the community to match its resources to its identified prioritized health problems better.

The third step outlined in Figure 7.2 is the major challenge of aligning providers, managers, and governing board members both within and across the medical, health, and larger community sectors. By alignment, we mean the development of a shared vision, values, agreed-on strategies and action plans, and financial incentives and rewards that promote cooperative behavior. This is often a tall order to fill even within each sector, let alone across sectors. It requires adept leadership deeply committed to the importance of community health improvement and willing to rise above parochial organizational interests; a strong input from key influential individuals and groups in the community; and the ability to create a sense of legitimacy—that is, a sense that what is being done is the right thing to do on the part of all involved. Our experience to date is that achieving internal alignment within each sector helps to facilitate alignment across sectors. Specifically, those who directly provide health and social services to community residents need to feel that they are supported by their management teams and that the governing board members in turn understand and support both management and those who directly provide the services. In brief, the "disconnects" between governance, management, and service delivery need to be minimized. To the extent that this is accomplished within each sector (for example, health care delivery, public health, education, and housing), it becomes easier for individuals at whatever level (governance, management, or service delivery) to interact across sectors because they know they have the support of others within their own sector and their own organization. The results are quicker decision making, more effective problem solving, and recognition of expanded opportunities for collaboration.

Once the building blocks are put in place, the community health care management system has the potential to operate the "capability wheel" shown in Figure 7.2. The community's desired health care end states drive the strategies and action plans. This involves articulating and implementing a "theory of action" (Patton, 1978) based on system thinking that begins with understanding the desired end state and working backward to identifying all of the actions required to achieve that state. The theory of action can also be viewed as a cause-and-effect logic map with a set of underlying assumptions. For example, a desired end state may be to reduce teenage pregnancy by 50 percent over three years. The steps necessary to do this might include appointing a task force with a representative from all groups that can affect the outcomes; developing a specific time frame with intermediate milestones to be achieved; providing needed resources; developing specific programs regarding sex and health education classes in schools; working with religious and youth organizations; developing a parent and peer counseling program; making birth control alternatives accessible; targeting special intervention strategies for highly susceptible subgroups; and so on. For some conditions such as asthma and diabetes, the theory of action may be codified in guidelines, protocols, and pathways based on evidence of how to achieve superior outcomes. The theory of action, of course, is seldom static but will need to be revised and refined as experience is gained with what works and does not work under various circumstances.

As shown in Figure 7.2, strategies and action plans influence and are influenced by the implementation of continuous improvement processes. These processes, originally applied in other sectors (Deming, 1986; Juran, 1989), have been used in health care delivery for over a decade (cf. Berwick, Godfrey, and Roessner, 1990; Blumenthal and Laffel, 1989, Sahney and Warden, 1991) with varying results (Shortell, Bennett, and Byck, 1998; Blumenthal and Kilo 1998). There has been little application of CQI approaches to date, however, to communitywide health improvement initiatives. Yet the potential for payoff is likely to be large given the need to coordinate highly interdependent work across different sectors. The comparative advantage of continuous improvement processes is for work that involves such high degrees of reciprocal interdependence (Thompson, 1967) in which what one person or group does depends on receiving information, resources, or "clients" from others, while what the other person or group does depends in turn on receiving such input from the original party. This kind of health improvement work cries out for the removal of unnecessary complexity, the reduction of unneeded variance in performance and results, the implementation of more standardized procedures and protocols, and tools to track variance reduction and resulting outcomes over time. For example, in the case of asthma, a registry-based care management system might be established along with a data system to track outcomes over time. A cause-and-effect diagram might identify key areas for attention. A protocol might be developed along with instructions for use by providers, patients, family members, schools, and others.

Continuous improvement processes, in turn, influence and are influenced by the results. To what extent is the incidence of teenage pregnancy, domestic violence, substance abuse, and hospitalizations for diabetes and asthma reduced? These outcomes form part of the new knowledge base regarding the end states for the identified problem and provide opportunities to raise the bar by setting even higher standards for achievement. This can be accomplished through the incorporation of new technologies and treatments, including increasing patient and family access to information.

As shown in Figure 7.2, the community health care management system capability wheel is anchored and driven in the middle by information systems. The lack of sufficiently well-developed information systems to identify problems, facilitate treatment and referral, and monitor progress and outcomes is the Achilles' heel of almost all community health improvement initiatives. Although some progress is being made by some health care delivery systems and community organizations, there is as yet little linkage of "medical care treatment"–based information systems to the information systems of community health and social service agencies. The issue is important and complex. The federal government needs to establish some definitional parameters and standards along with dealing with privacy and confidentiality protection issues. To the extent that this can be achieved, private sector firms can then compete within the established regulatory framework to develop the needed systems. A second generation of community health information networks (CHINs) may offer one approach to the problem.

## Organization and Core Functions of the Community Health Care Management System

Within each community, the community health care management system (CHCMS) might be organized along the lines of local security and exchange commissions as quasi-administrative and publicly accountable bodies. As suggested by Figure 7.2, the CHCMS would be charged with responsibility for three major core functions:

1. Assessing the health status of the community and, in so doing, identifying and prioritizing the health needs of the community

2. Developing and implementing strategies and action plans for addressing these needs by organizing the community's assets, resources, competencies, and capabilities to do so

3. Being held clinically and fiscally accountable for results to relevant political bodies

The CHCMS would make an annual report to the relevant political body—for example, the mayor's office, city manager's office, or county supervisor. This report would also be made available to the community at large via newspaper, television, radio, and the Internet. An example of such a report for the State of Wisconsin is shown in Figure 7.3.

This suggested organization and functioning of the CHCMS is well within the experience of many communities throughout the United States. For example, the American Hospital Association/Health Research and Educational Trust Community Care Network (CCN) Demonstration Program, which involved over 250 applicants, 60 finalists, and 25 awardees, is based on four underlying dimensions: (1) community health focus, (2) delivering a seamless continuum of care, (3) managing within limited resources, and (4) being accountable to the community (Bogue, Antia, Harmata, and Hall, 1997). These are essentially identical to the three core functions of the CHCMS outlined above. In fact, the funded CCN sites represent twenty-five specific examples of evolving CHCMSs in their respective communities.

The study systems also provide evidence of a readiness to implement the community health care management concept. For example, all but one of the systems already has an organized approach to community health improvement, with a specific designated budget, staff, and leadership. Between 1 and approximately 8 percent of the operating budgets of each system was committed to community health initiatives. Every system had an organized program for the uninsured and medically indigent and also for senior citizens. All but one system had an organized school health program. Seven of the nine systems had organized programs directed at reducing teenage pregnancy and domestic violence, and had externally funded demonstration projects to improve community health that ranged from $1.5 million per year to $12.0 million per year. Six of the nine systems had organized programs addressing substance abuse. Some, such as Fairview, issue an annual community health partnership report. Fairview's report states:

> Community relationships and the regions served by Fairview Community Health are called Partnerships. The criteria include having a defined mission, vision, and membership, as well as clearly defined goals and objectives. Fairview provides staff, resources, and facilitation of Partnership activities to support community ownership of the goals of creating healthier communities.

The report card goes on to summarize sixty-four partnership initiatives.

### Key Success Factors for Community Health Care Management Systems

The more successful community health care management systems are likely to be differentiated from the less successful on seven factors: breadth of organizational membership, leadership depth, sharing the winner's circle, managing and channeling conflict, recognizing life cycles, the ability to "patch," and the ability to track progress with information systems.

Figure 7.3.  Annual Wisconsin Population Health Checkup.

| Population Health Indicators | Data for fifty states | | |
|---|---|---|---|
| **Health Outcomes** | **Highest** | **Wisconsin** | **Lowest** |
| Age-adjusted adult respiratory disease deaths per 100,000 persons, 1994 | 182.6 | 115.0 | 78.9 |
| AIDS cases per 100,000 persons, 1995 | 69.2 | 7.2 | 1.1 |
| Age-adjusted deaths per 100,000 persons, 1994 | 988.4 | 778.6 | 655.6 |
| Age-adjusted motor vehicle accident deaths per 100,000 persons, 1994 | 32.3 | 15.0 | 7.5 |
| Percentage of live births low birthweight, 1993 | 10% | 6% | 5% |
| Age-adjusted suicide deaths per 100,000 persons, 1994 | 23.7 | 12.0 | 7.1 |
| Average days in past month physical health "not good," 1994 | 3.8 | 2.9 | 2.2 |
| **Behavioral Factors** | | | |
| Births to teens as percent of live births, 1993 | 21% | 10% | 7% |
| Percentage of population using safety belts, 1994 | 84% | 64% | 32% |
| Percentage of adults who smoke, 1994 | 29% | 23% | 16% |
| Percentage of adults overweight, 1994 | 32% | 30% | 20% |
| Percentage of adults (age 18+) who drink and drive, 1993 | 5% | 5% | 1% |
| Percentage of adults who binge drink 1993 | 23% | 23% | 4% |

*Source:* Libby and others (1997).

| Healthiest States | Wisconsin's rank among 50 states | | | Least Healthy States |
|---|---|---|---|---|
| 1 | 10 | 25 | 40 | 50 |
| UT  4 | | | | NV |
| ND | 10 | | | NY |
| HI | 13 | | | MS |
| RI | 15 | | | MS |
| AK | 16 | | | MS |
| NJ | 18 | | | WY |
| KS | | 29 | | WV |
| NH | 12 | | | MS |
| HI | | 24 | | RI |
| UT | | 27 | | NV |
| HI | | | 47 | MS |
| MD | | | | 50 WI |
| TN | | | | 50 WI |
| | 10 | 25 | 40 | 50 |

Wisconsin's rank among 50 states

### Breadth of Organizational Membership

The size and composition of the CHCMS organizational membership base will vary as a function of the number and breadth of problems a community wishes to address. In general, however, a broader
membership base reflecting a greater number of sectors (such as public health, education, religious organizations, law enforcement,
housing, transportation, environment, hospitals, health systems,
and physician groups) is likely to be more effective than a smaller,
narrower base of organizations. This is because most community
health improvement issues are pervasive in their impact and require
the concerted coordinated action of many sectors for resolution. In
the CCN program, the number of organizational members increased
from an average of ten from the first year to twenty-two by the end
of the third year, reflecting the recognition of the need for additional partners to achieve identified community health improvement objectives. This, of course, does not mean that each member
participates in the same way. For example, the CCN partnerships
had three categories of membership:

- Full working partners, who provided financial resources
  and/or staff and committed considerable time and energy to the partnership's activities.

- Participating partners, who typically participated actively in meetings to develop strategies and plans but
  were less involved than the full working partners.

- Informing partners, who did not directly provide resources or develop strategies or plans but were kept informed of progress and were willing to offer support as
  needed. They typically provided additional legitimacy
  to the CCN's efforts.

The two underlying principles in forming these categories were
to recognize the comparative advantage and interest of each party
and to be inclusive rather than exclusive.

## Leadership Depth

CHCMSs built on the leadership of a single or even a few individuals are not likely to endure in the long run, for at least four reasons. First, it is often the case that leaders who are superb in getting efforts launched are less effective as maintainers or long-run builders of the effort. Different preferences, interests, and skill sets are involved at each stage of development. Second, the problems and challenges faced by partnerships such as those represented by the CHCMS concept change over time, and no single individual possesses all of the necessary skills, insights, or foresight to adapt to these changes. Third, leaders burn out. Fourth, leaders sometimes leave their positions or even the community altogether. As a result, it is important to build depth of leadership within the CHCMS and, ideally, across sectors. Different individuals are needed at different points in time. This is consistent with the principle of subsidiarity used by some Catholic health care systems: that the group closest to the problem should deal with it, receiving support from higher-level groups as necessary.

## Sharing the Winner's Circle

The CHCMS is a complex set of interorganizational relationships that requires extensive collaboration and coordination as well as subordination of individual organizational interests to achieve a larger common good. As such, effective leaders realize that the "winning" and "getting credit" needs to be spread around. Effective leaders figure out what organizations need to win at given points in time for the community overall to benefit. At some point it may be the health department, at another point the school, and at still another point the local hospital or health system. A useful analogy is that of bicycle team racing. It is a team sport that allows for different individual members of the team to win or "lead" on any given day or leg of the race. Each member has to do some of the "grunt" work ("blocking" and "drafting," for example) to help the designated "lead" for that day. In a successful CHCMS, the dynamics are much the same.

## Managing and Channeling Conflict

Partnerships associated with the CHCMS concept are likely to be sufficiently diverse as to create great need for reconciling and channeling conflicting perspectives that will arise—both about what to do and how to do it. It is important that the decision-making process be perceived as fair and open, and as fact filled and data oriented as possible. Everyone should be encouraged to arrive at the best solution. It is important that discussions stay focused on the issue and the objectives to be achieved rather than on personalities. Decisions and events must be placed within a long-run context rather than merely focused on short-run issues. Ways must be found to enlarge the playing field rather than to see all decisions from a win-lose perspective. It is important to emphasize how the community will benefit in the long run even though some parties may be disadvantaged in the short run. And it is important to follow up with those who may be "hurt" by a decision to explain that this was not the intent, to express appreciation for everyone's input, and to encourage continued involvement.

Evidence from the evaluation of the CCN Demonstration Program suggests that these approaches were successful in preventing destructive conflict from developing and in channeling conflict in positive directions. Serious conflicts are particularly likely to arise as the CHCMSs tackle the tougher health problems in the community involving the need for one or more organizational members to delete or consolidate services or reduce staff, with all the attendant financial implications. It may also be that the toughest problems to address are those of intermediate difficulty. Relatively easy problems can be taken care of in a relatively straightforward fashion or simply allocated among organizational members of the partnership. Everyone recognizes that extremely difficult problems require a high degree of cooperative and collaborative effort, even if individual parties may need to make sacrifices. However, with problems of intermediate severity, it is not clear whether a given organization can handle the problem or potentially competing organizations. It is in these areas that the ability to manage and channel the conflict is particularly important.

### Recognizing Life Cycles; Handing off the Baton

Effective CHCMSs will learn to recognize the naturally occurring life cycles of an organization well documented in the literature (Kimberly, 1980; D'Aunno and Zuckerman, 1987). These are typically described in terms of the start-up stage, early growth and development stage, maturity stage, and the decline or renewal stage. It is important to recognize that not only will the CHCMS have an internal life cycle dynamic but that the health issues selected to be addressed will also have a life cycle, as will the larger community of which the CHCMS is a part. For example, a newly started CHCMS may be embedded within the third term of an important public official or dominant political structure. In reverse fashion, a newly elected group of community political leaders can reenergize a CHCMS that has lost steam or is bogged down in internecine warfare. To deal with these issues frequently requires different leadership at different times. A CHCMS must have the wisdom of knowing when to pass the baton, to recognize when someone else needs to step up to the plate, and to develop a strong bench of "pinch hitters." To continue the mixed metaphor, successful CHCMSs need to be both good at running relays and pinching hitting for each other.

### Ability to "Patch"

In the business strategy literature, "patching" refers to the ability to remap business units to match rapidly changing market demands (Eisenhardt and Brown, 1999). It is particularly important in rapidly changing industries where agility is required. Examples are Dell, Intel, Microsoft, and 3M. In the context of a CHCMS, it refers to the ability of the partnership to remap or reposition the assets, resources, competencies, and capabilities of the community to address changing health care needs and priorities and evolving political, social, regulatory, and economic forces. For example, delivering cancer screening services to rural Hispanic women requires strategies and a set of resources very different from addressing substance abuse among teenagers, increasing child immunization rates, or developing a secondary prevention program for cardiovascular disease. As progress is made in one or more of these areas, attention needs to turn to other areas involving a reconfiguration of resources and strategies. Hospitals may play a lead role in some of these efforts, and no role in others. The same holds for the health department, schools, physician practices, and so on. Instability in the environment—turnover among key community leaders, mergers of hospitals, cutbacks in state or federal funding, or introduction of new legislation—also necessitates the need to patch.

CHCMSs that lack the ability to patch are less likely to sustain themselves than those that acquire this capability. It is, of course, also related to the breadth of membership of the CHCMS. The greater the breadth, the greater is the potential ability to patch.

## Information Systems: Ability to Track Progress

The final key success factor for CHCMSs is the ability to track progress on their objectives for purposes of internal continuous improvement and the ability to make adjustments for external accountability to the community. This is a major challenge and impediment to achieving community health improvement objectives. A major objective for CHCMSs should be to establish an information infrastructure that will serve their internal and external needs. A cross-site, cross-sector task force should be established to agree on data needs, define terms and standards, explore platforms and software, and consider the needs of multiple stakeholders. Shared internal funding as well as external funding will be needed. Progress in building the information infrastructure will be slow but must be sustained. At the same time, what is eventually needed must not be the enemy of what can be done now. Successful CHCMSs will do everything they can to increase the visibility of data, information and feedback on implementation, and success of their action plans for improving community health.

## Major Challenges to the CHCMS Concept

It is difficult enough for individual organizations to succeed in today's demanding, and even punishing, health care environment. To ask these organizations to work with other organizations to improve community health and well-being that may or may not directly or even indirectly benefit one's own organization in the short or long run is a tall order. Each organization has its own mission, strategies, plans, resources, and stakeholders to whom it is accountable. The governing board of the organization has its own fiduciary responsibility to preserve and enhance the institution's assets. Thus, appropriately, each health care organization should ask how participation in a community health care management system benefits the organization? "What is in it for my own organization?" is a valid question.

But it is also the case that most health and social service organizations have explicitly indicated in their mission statements that they "strive to promote the health of individuals and the communities at large" or "to meet the health needs of the community" or variations on these words. The real question is whether each organization views accomplishment of its own objectives as constituting that contribution to "community health and well-being" *or* whether it sees its organization as part of a larger interdependent network needed to have an important impact on the health of the community. This is the largest challenge facing the CHCMS concept in the United States.

The operating principles of U.S. culture are centered on individualism as opposed to the more collective orientations of Canada and Western European nations (Bellah and others, 1998). We tend to favor autonomy over solidarity, individual choice over collective determination, and specialization over integration. Our individualistic orientation has largely served us well. But as we said in the first edition of this book, we may have lost the ability to achieve balance on these dimensions. We have accumulated large amounts of individual capital, but perhaps at the expense of social capital. Before the CHCMS can succeed, we must begin to pay more attention to investments in social capital, "such as the networks, norms, and trust that facilitate coordination and cooperation for mutual benefits" (Putnam, 1993, p. 35).

There appears to be renewed interest in community building and the communitarian approach to social advancement (Bellah and others, 1998; Etzioni, 1999). Nonetheless, the application of the communitarian perspective to the health care sector appears complex and ambiguous. U.S. health care policymakers appear to have little faith in using communities to allocate health care resources, particularly for medical care, although apparently less so for issues involving long-term care, substance abuse, AIDS, and related conditions (Schlesinger, 1997). This may be due in part to a distrust of large medical institutions, which often have viewed the community as an object to be worked on or as a means of support for individual interests instead of as a collaborating partner to improve health (Schlesinger, 1997). The role that these large institutions, particularly organized delivery systems, can play within the context of the CHCMS is addressed in the following section.

## Organized Delivery Systems and the Challenge of Integrated Health Care

In the earlier edition of this book, we noted that organized delivery systems are ideally characterized by holographic properties in which the *system* is represented in each of its constituent parts: hospitals, physician groups, long-term care facilities, divisions, departments, service lines, task forces, committees, and individuals. Holographic properties exist in a symbiotic relationship with integrative processes. Integration is the process by which actions are formed, coordinated, or blended into a functioning or unified whole. It is an essential process in building a holographic organization because before the whole can be embedded in each part, it must first exist as a "whole"—that is, something must be brought together from different elements. For example, in order for diabetic patients to receive the same quality of care from physician group A within a system as they would from physician group B (that is, for the whole to be in each part), the nature of what constitutes high-quality "holistic" diabetic care needs to be defined and implemented. This might be done, for example, through the development of guidelines and protocols that stipulate how a variety of steps are to be executed and in what order. Disease management or overall case and care management systems will play a similar role. The result is a whole that can be implanted in each of the system. Thus, integration is both a cause and an effect of a holographic organization. It is a cause in that certain elements, processes, and activities must be coordinated with each other to create wholes. And it is also an effect because as the whole is reflected in each part, the parts give rise to greater integration potential with other parts of the system. A well-integrated part has greater carrying capacity to link up and energize other parts of the system and thereby create greater value.

The organized delivery system's role within the larger CHCMS is to extend its holographic properties to embrace the creation, maintenance, and enhancement of the health of the community beyond the delivery of health care services. The goal of the organized delivery system is to promote and defend the health of its defined population. To achieve this, it needs to expand its carrying capacity to include a larger range of organizations in the community that influence health. An example of such an extension is shown in Figure 7.4 using Group Health/Kaiser Permanente's Population Health Management model. As indicated in this model, promoting population-based health requires a focus on five stages, ranging from presymptomatic to end-of-life care. The greatest value is created by keeping people in the presymptomatic state. If organized delivery systems were paid for

Figure 7.4. Group Health/Kaiser-Permanente Population Health Management Model Extension.

| | | | FIVE STAGES | | |
|---|---|---|---|---|---|
| | 1<br>Presymptomatic | 2<br>Symptomatic | 3<br>Acute | 4<br>Chronic | 5<br>End of Life |
| Community<br>Health-Building<br>Activities | | | | | |
| Health Status Assessment | • Community<br>  organizations<br>• Health<br>  department<br>• Hospitals and<br>  health systems | | | | |
| Demand Management<br>Disease Prevention<br>and Health Promotion | • Jobs<br>• Housing<br>• Education<br>• Environment<br>• Family support<br>• Law enforcement<br>• Health care providers<br>• Health department<br>• Hospitals and<br>  health systems<br>• Internet | | | | |

Self-care Management

- Internet
- Family support
- Jobs
- Housing
- Education
- Environment
- Religious organizations
- Health professionals
- Hospitals and health systems

Professional Disease Management

- Physicians and other health professionals
- Hospitals and health systems
- Long-term care and rehabilitation facilities
- Internet
- Family support
- Religious organizations
- Housing
- Environment

keeping their populations healthy, incentives would be created for "front-loading" activities associated with demand management through a variety of disease prevention and health promotion activities. These would emphasize the importance of clean air and water, recreational facilities, education, jobs, housing, transportation, law enforcement, family support services, and the role of religious organizations. Organized delivery systems would play a facilitating and supportive role in working with these organizations to prevent illness and disability and enhance health. Estimates are that preventable illness makes up approximately 90 percent of the burden of illness and its associated costs (U.S. Public Health Service, 1991).

Over time, of course, community residents will develop symptoms and require various acute care, chronic care, and end-of-life services. In these stages, the organized delivery system will assume greater responsibility for restoring and enhancing health and dealing with the burden of illness. Value is created here by restoring these individuals to their maximum state of functioning as quickly as possible. This too requires closer integration between the organized delivery system and the other organizations shown in Figure 7.4, particularly in regard to secondary prevention activities related to diet, exercise, promotion of self-efficacy, home support services, and a safe environment.

By creating greater interdependence between organized delivery systems and community organizations, the groundwork is laid for an exchange of holographic properties between the two sets. As financial resources, staff, and technologies are shared, more of the broad-based community perspective on creation of health becomes embedded within the organized delivery system, while more of the holographic properties of the organized delivery system become embedded within the community organizations. The AHA/HRET Community Care Network Demonstration Program is an example as the community-based organizations have learned from the organized delivery systems regarding managing under limited resources and ways of using guidelines and protocols to achieve a more seamless continuum of care. In return, the organized delivery systems have learned how better to focus on community health issues and to participate in mutual forums of accountability with the community. The net result of such initiatives within the context of the community health care management system is an increased capacity to deal with complex health problems in the community and an increased capability to adapt to change.

## The Organized Delivery System Challenge

The discussion is this chapter is largely what *might be true* and is largely theoretical. Creating integrated systems of community health promotion, maintenance, and enhancement is a daunting task requiring vision, commitment, skills, persistence, resilience, and good fortune. Figure 7.5 depicts the challenges in terms of the analogy of driving a nail—in this case, the nail of health improvement. The underlying concept is one of alignment. Funding and

Figure 7.5.  Driving the Nail of Health Improvement.

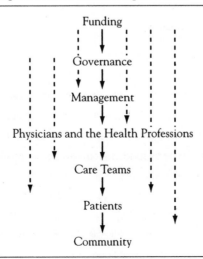

payment systems must provide the incentives for the governance and management of community health systems to develop focused strategies that can be implemented by physicians and health care teams to meet patient and community needs. If any one of these drivers is off center, the nail begins to go sideways. As a nation, we are not even close to driving this nail straight despite the best of intentions on the part of many groups.

In the short term, we are not optimistic that much progress will be made. There are too many negative forces. When it comes to public policy and health care policy in particular, the United States favors incrementalism. The best that we can hope for is that the leadership, determination, and persistence of a few will serve as a platform and beacon for others if or when the policy environment becomes more favorable for providing integrated health care delivery. In this regard, the words of Max Planck (1948) may prove prophetic: "A new scientific truth does not triumph by convincing its opponents and making them see the light but rather because its opponents eventually die, and a new generation grows up that is familiar with the new truth." The same may be true for achieving the ultimate potential of organized delivery systems.

### Mercy Health Services

Mercy Health Services has identified its top goal in its systemwide Fiscal Year 1998–2000 Strategic Plan to "continuously improve community health through community partnerships and advocacy, focusing on populations-at-risk." This is the first of six strategic objectives for that planning period which locates this objective under "Community Partnerships." The second objective relates to growth and the remaining four to quality and value.

The first strategic objective derives directly from the third element of Mercy's Fiscal Year 1998–2000 Vision Statement: "We Will Use Our System's Growing Strength to Improve Community Health and to Serve and Advocate for Populations-at-Risk."

Under this strategic plan, it is expected that 100 percent of Mercy's Community Health Care Systems (CHCS) or local operating units will be "facilitating/participating in community partnerships programs addressing broad-based community health status indicators." Examples include immunization rates, smoking rates, substance abuse, domestic violence, and economic opportunities.

Mercy organized the Community Health Status Priority Team of almost thirty people from throughout the Mercy system and commissioned it to conduct a review of community health improvement activities. (There are only a few priority teams, and they are used only to address the largest issues.) The goal of the team was generally to "adopt new community health improvement partnerships models using best practices in Mercy Health Services (MHS) and other organizations." The team identified the following tasks for it to conduct:

- Inventorying existing community health care systems (CHCS) work to understand individual capabilities

- Developing process and structure for sharing expertise across the system

- Developing a framework for strategic indicators and targets

- Leveraging system strength for opportunity development and further assisting with the realignment of Strategic Initiatives for the Poor (SIP) programs to improve outcomes and positively impact health status

- Developing strategies to increase MHS advocacy efforts at the local, state, and national levels

## Progress Toward Community Health Improvement Involvement

At Mercy considerable community involvement has historically been fostered by its long-standing SIP program, which was formalized in 1988 and always included both target groups: the poor and the general community. During 1998, for example, Mercy spent $94 million to fund SIP programs that encompassed traditional charity care, treatment of Medicaid recipients, and population-at-risk programs such as immunization clinics for at-risk, poor children. Mercy's efforts for the general community include treatment of Medicare beneficiaries, education and research, and community service programs such as St. Joseph Mercy-Oakland's Caring for Aging Parents program, which is available to anyone regardless of economic status.

A further step in the evolution of this kind of program is being taken through an important strategic objective that expands this involvement to the improvement of overall community health status indicators in existing service areas. The Priority Team indicated that to move forward in this direction, Mercy would need to secure strong commitments from both management and governance and work with other community-based entities in a partnership style.

Initially, operating units completed a survey to document existing community health improvement programs throughout the system. A pattern emerged from the survey results that allowed a categorization of existing programs in the following ways:

- Broad-based "healthy communities" programs.
- Programs targeting a major at-risk subset population of a community.
- Other special community initiatives.

The Priority Team came up with a number of recommendations for action:

- Incorporating specific commitments to community health status improvement within each CHCS strategic plan
- Promoting active CHCS governance involvement in the development of these plans and specific follow-up activities within the community
- Establishing a supportive "intelligent network" within MHS to share learnings and to promote healthier community development

- Developing within each CHCS a set of quantitative community-specific health status indicators

- Adopting one selected systemwide community health improvement initiative for special systemwide support, including fundraising

- Considering MHS communitywide health status partnership initiatives as a complement to and in no way a replacement for SIP

- Requiring the new Healthier Communities Affinity Group to develop further specific recommendations for an expanded overall MHS advocacy program for community health status improvement

The work of the Priority Team provided a good start to a refocused and enhanced SIP program. However, there are some barriers limiting its development.

## Obstacles and Barriers to Community Health Improvement Involvement

One of the major barriers to progress in implementing the varied recommendations of the Priority Team is the lack of focused leadership to take the helm on this project. This is due mainly to ongoing discussions of the pending major merger with another multistate health system, which has frozen the position of director of social accountability and community service for the entire system.

Given the lack of focused leadership, there has been little progress on one of the more challenging barriers: lack of specified performance indicators for all programs and activities at both the local service level and systemwide. Without these measures, an appropriate evolution of these programs from a planning sense is very difficult.

In addition, Michigan is experiencing a confusing and poorly funded Medicaid payment environment. In the conservative political environment, the policy is to reduce Medicaid expenditures by a variety of changing mechanisms, including attempting to have existing providers pick up the slack for a state that is systematically reducing the numbers of Medicaid recipients without providing alternative coverage.

Further, in the provider marketplace, "health status" does not have a lot of appeal in the face of strong supply-side competition that is not being fought out over improvement of health status in the community but rather on maintaining or enhancing an economic position.

Finally, having a program in place that already meets some of the goals of a revised community health improvement program provides a sort of internal inertia. Since the SIP has been in place for over ten years, there is not a desperate need to correct a terrible deficiency but rather an opportunity to move this program beyond its focus on remedial services to the poor to preventive and other services for the whole community.

## Keys to Success

The "inventory subgroup" of the Priority Team systematically solicited detailed information from each of the many programs involved in community health improvement across the Mercy System. From this they identified some of the key elements:

"Strong community vision that drives the goal setting" (Creating a Healthier Macomb).

"Allowing and encouraging other organizations besides Mercy to take lead in various initiatives" (Healthy Dubuque, 2000).

"Program success is defined at the individual, family, and community levels" (Healthy Start/Healthy Families Oakland).

"The 13 member coalition, partnering together to tackle this complex social issue, will be a key success factor, as no single agency can address this issue alone" (Washtenaw Housing Alliance).

"Determine baseline outcome measurement prior to launching program" (Derek Edwards Bike Safety Program).

"Establishment of a Seniors Advisory Board" (Senior Services Health Clinic at Burnham Brooks Senior Center).

"Target physicians first" (Partnership for Immunizations, Battle Creek).

"Availability of flexible funding to allow creativity in the approaches to the problem" (Teen Sexuality: Choices and Consequences).

"Addressing root causes of a number of health issues simultaneously—like substance abuse." (Healthy Tomorrows, North Iowa).

## Lessons Learned

The Improving Community Health Status Priority Team culled numerous lessons learned from its inventory and identified the following common themes:

- Facilitate, do not dominate.
- Relationship building with community groups is essential; this requires time and perseverance.
- Adopt a broader definition of health than the medical model.
- Establish baseline and outcomes measures in concert with the community; a community's definition of health problems may be very different from those of providers; minimize preconceived notions.
- Broad-based community and funding support can be obtained with hard work and appropriate approaches.
- Use and build on existing efforts of community organizations and agencies where possible.

One agency in Muskegon showed a particular insight that might be helpful to many:

"Don't take it personally; nobody trusts hospital management. They think we are better organized and run than we are and it is intimidating to many. Do not be afraid to show vulnerability and admit ignorance" (Family Coordinating Council)."

## Future Directions

The future of community health improvement activities at Mercy is currently tied up in the new position for overall director of social accountability and community service for the entire system, which is on hold pending strategic activity with another health system. But it is clear that Mercy and its partners will continue to provide extensive programming in this area in keeping with its mission: "We work together and with others, in the tradition of the Sisters of Mercy, to relieve suffering of body, mind and spirit and to improve the health of our communities."

•    •    •    •    •    •

## Sutter Health

Toward the end of June 1999, the senior vice president for public affairs at Sutter Health, headquartered in Sacramento, California, sent a thick binder, entitled *Community Benefit Resource Guide,* to "affiliate community benefit planners," "affiliate social accountability reporters," and "affiliate communications professionals" across the entire Sutter Health system. The purpose was to provide a tool for guidance in the development of future community benefit activities locally. Part of the reason for sending this information was to note the requirements under California's Community Benefit Law (SB 697). More important, it was to emphasize that "Community Benefit is critical to advancing our not-for-profit mission and has been highlighted as a priority initiative in the 1999–2001 Strategic Plan." Sutter Health had engaged in extensive community benefit activities before the law went into place in 1995 and continues to exceed its requirements.

## Progress Toward Community Health Improvement Involvement

Although Sutter has been directly engaged in community benefit activities for a long time, these activities continue to evolve. One of the challenges is to become more sophisticated in defining and measuring community benefit. This requires some reeducation about what it means internally. To do this, Sutter has undertaken systemwide training in community benefits and put everybody on a common software system to track community benefits activities. Moreover, it has made sure that everybody in the system is "doing the right thing" in terms of defining community benefit by tightening the definitions of this kind of activity and in the past two years has included community benefits in local CEOs' performance criteria.

Since 1998 Sutter has participated in the Voluntary Hospital Association's community health improvement network (CHIN). This affiliation helps provide education and tools on how to improve community health improvement methods and move programs toward sustainability. Sutter personnel attend CHIN conferences to explore new ideas and learn from successes elsewhere and bring this information back to share internally.

In 1998, Sutter invested over $2 million in all forms of community benefit activity, which required over 8 percent of net patient revenue from the entire system. An internal community benefits inventory showed that Sutter Health and its affiliates offered over eighty-five programs to provide access to health education and basic medical services.

Beyond traditional charity care and unpaid costs of public programs, these other community benefit activities include nonbilled services, such as many different types of community education and outreach including the Health Academy with the San Juan School District; medical education and research for providers at all levels of training; subsidized health services such as the collaborative effort to care for the indigent at primary care clinics in Sacramento County and also with the Yolo Health Alliance; cash and in-kind donations, including equipment donation and food to shelters and hunger programs; and community-building activities ranging from physical improvements through graffiti removal and street lighting to support of child care cooperatives. Some of these programs require minimal resources and mainly provide opportunities for "good citizen" collaboration. Others, like the Yolo Health Alliance, are carried out as a partnership with Yolo County, Communicare Clinics, and Sutter and require a substantial ongoing support at the level of $250,000 per year.

The immediate reasons for becoming involved in these many activities are just as varied as the activities themselves. One stimulus was the deep economic recession of the early 1990s, which caused Sacramento County to cut back on its primary care programs for the indigent. Sutter Health along with Mercy Health Care and other partners recognized that this was creating a large and crucial gap in services and stepped forward with significant financial and in-kind services to help minimize the impact of local government cutbacks. Both systems also realized that providing upstream resources in terms of preventive and primary care is less costly than care provided in their emergency departments later. An attempt is made to ensure that all of the community benefit activities are focused on Sutter's key strategic direction of providing improved access to care, especially for women and children, on their own and with other nonprofit providers within their service area.

## Obstacles and Barriers to Community Health Improvement Involvement

The obstacles or barriers to encouraging involvement in community health improvement activities are many. First, Sutter covers a large geographic area in northern California, which includes a number of diverse communities. No single program or even set of programs is likely to meet the local needs in each of those places. Flexibility is required to encourage activities that meet local needs while incorporating reporting mechanisms that allow for the strategic use of systemwide information about community benefit activities.

Measurement is a challenge with many kinds of community benefit activities. It requires selecting and implementing measures of impact, as well as elaborating cost-benefit justifications for these activities in a constrained resource environment where programs sometimes face off against one another.

In some cases, there are distinct financial challenges for a local affiliate (hospital facility). Community benefits activities are mainly decentralized throughout the system, and the resources for community benefit come out of the local budget. For some affiliates that are more cash strapped than others, the question comes up: Do you lay off personnel or do you cut back community benefit programs? Sutter is looking for partners in some of its service areas where resources are tight or where significant leverage can be obtained from bringing another health or social service provider into the situation. The central (corporate) budget for community benefits is mainly for staffing and for limited discretionary funds for small project support anywhere in the system.

In some service areas where Sutter operates, collaboration with competitors can be an obstacle. In other areas, such as the Sacramento area in the Eastern Division, there is significant and useful collaboration on needs assessment, planning, and some joint activities. For example, in the Sacramento area, Sutter collaborates with Kaiser, the University of California at Davis Medical Center, and Mercy Health on a comprehensive regional needs assessment called the Healthy Community Forum.

Another obstacle to community health improvement activities is a common understanding of what community benefits is all about. There has been a general failure to communicate information regarding Sutter's "good works" to the public, which has allowed Sutter to be seen as a provider of "corporate health care" and limits public input.

Although there are new foundations in California that are specialized in providing resources to programs within the state, they have not been major funders for Sutter's community benefits activities. This may be due both to the fact that these foundations are new and finding their way in terms of identifying worthwhile investments and the "corporate" image of Sutter Health. Regardless of the source, financial resources are needed if community benefits activities are to move forward.

## Keys to Success

The keys to success for community benefits activities involve both "CEO leadership" from the top of Sutter and local initiative from each of their service areas. Support from the top is clearly evident through various communications by the board of trustees and top management, the inclusion of community benefits goals in the systemwide strategic plan, and the inclusion of the executive responsible for systemwide community benefits coordination in the top management team. This team is made up of nine executives plus the CEO.

The senior vice president for public affairs at Sutter Health has convened a "Community Benefits Council" from across the system. These twenty to thirty people meet quarterly to brainstorm and share best practices. These activities help encourage creativity among the members, refine the definition of community benefits activities, and provide an opportunity for managers to discuss ways to make sure that community benefits get to and stay on the top agenda of local service area CEOs.

The 1995 legislation that requires tax-exempt hospitals in California to provide information related to the community benefits they provide establishes expectations for a focus on community benefits activities. However some systems, such as Sutter's, would prefer clearer definitions regarding community benefits and more refined reporting requirements. Because there are no formal state definitions of community benefit, it is not possible to compare performance across systems.

Another key to success involves communication from local service area CEOs. In 1997, a systemwide requirement was implemented that CEOs include community benefits on their individual list of management objectives. In order to facilitate this evolution, several systemwide venues were used to emphasize the importance of community benefits, including a keynote spot in the governance symposium for all trustees in the system in 1997 (reinforced by a breakout session in 1998), as well as a keynote spot in the 1997 management symposium (reinforced by breakout sessions in 1998 and 1999 at the same annual event).

## Lessons Learned

Although Sutter's community benefits activity is still evolving, some of the lessons it has learned can be shared with other systems:

- CEO leadership both centrally and locally has been very important.

- Explicit connection of community health improvement activities to system strategic and operational goals in the written strategic plan is very useful in conveying the importance of these activities.

- Local input from communities and local management from Sutter affiliates is essential.

- Information reporting requirements should be kept short and simple.

- In order to avoid undermining local initiative and responsiveness, limited systemwide standardization has been undertaken and wholesale centralization of these activities avoided.

- It is necessary to continuously put out the message of the importance of community benefits activities through various channels in the system.

## Future Directions

The senior vice president for public affairs at Sutter Health is enthusiastic about future opportunities to do more measurements in a more sophisticated way so that the organization can link community benefits activities with clinical initiatives.

At this point, Sutter's information systems, like those of so many other health systems, are limited. The result is that it has not been able to determine how many children it has immunized in the past year, let alone how immunization rates in Sutter service areas compare to immunization rates in other parts of the state. Nor can it determine exactly how many people are served by its community benefits activities because some affiliates track that information and some do not.

Sutter has begun installing tracking software across the system to help gather service information and develop the capacity to track progress toward accomplishment of Healthy People 2000–type goals. With additional information will come the opportunity to improve measuring systems and provide some justification for the merit of community health enhancement activities.

# Resource A

. . . . . . . . . . . . . . . . . . . . . . . . . . . . . . . .

## Methods and Measures

The original study involved extensive collection of both primary and secondary data over a period of four years, complemented by two summers of fieldwork involving on-site interviews with systems participants. Although efforts to update information for this new edition were not as extensive, much new information was collected during spring and summer 1999 in order to understand the current status of the systems that are featured here. These systems were: Advocate Health Care (Oak Brook, Illinois); Baylor Health Care System (Dallas, Texas); Fairview Health System (Minneapolis, Minnesota); Franciscan Health System (Tacoma, Washington); Henry Ford Health System (Detroit, Michigan); Mercy Health Services (Farmington Hills, Michigan); Sentara Healthcare (Norfolk, Virginia); Sisters of Providence (Seattle, Washington); and Sutter Health (Sacramento, California). Systems provided updated written materials, including the system's profile (an inventory of operating units), organizational structure (including organization charts), annual report, strategic plan, audited financial report, mission and vision statement, summary of physician groups, and summary of managed care efforts. Systems also provided information on their community health improvement efforts.

In addition to the written materials, key system leaders were surveyed in the summer of 1999 regarding the current status of functional, physician, and clinical integration efforts at their systems.

Those typically surveyed were the system's chief executive officer, chief operating officer, vice president–strategic planning/system development, chief financial officer, and top physician leader. Representatives from seven of the nine systems returned questionnaires. The actual average number of respondents per system was 4.0.

Functional integration covered the following functions, services, and elements: human resources, administrative support services, strategic planning, marketing, financial management–resource allocation, financial management–operating policies, information services, quality assurance and improvement, and promoting a shared culture.

The physician arrangements and activities included under physician integration were independent practice association, closed physician hospital organization, open physician hospital organization, management services organization, medical foundation, equity model physician group, salaried model physician group, joint venture, managed care contracting, physician credentialing, physician profiling, quality and outcome reporting, physician leadership development training programs, and physician recruitment.

Clinical integration included the following items and activities: development and implementation of clinical guidelines, protocols, and pathways; common patient medical record ID number; case management systems; disease state management models and approaches; demand management models and approaches; implementation of population-based community health assessments; clinical information systems to coordinate care of patients; continuous quality improvement project teams focused on inpatient processes; continuous quality improvement project teams focused on outpatient/primary care processes; inpatient clinical service line management; clinical service line management that covers both inpatient and outpatient; and quality improvement steering councils or equivalent.

For each of the functions, items, and activities, the system leaders were asked how that particular item was provided, that is, (1) each unit had/did its own; (2) the function/service element was shared by two or more operating units/service lines within the system; (3) regional or divisional offices provided the function/service/element; and/or (4) the system provided the function/service/element for all operating units. Respondents could check as many of these as applied. These system leaders were also asked to assess how important integration of this function/service/element was for the system's plans, from not very important (1) to very important (3). Respondents were also asked the degree to which they were satisfied with the current status of the function/service/element across the system, from not satisfied at all (1) to very satisfied (5). Finally, for functional integration, the system leaders were asked to what extent the integration of each function/service/element was proceeding on the system's timetable, from behind over twelve months (1) to within one month of schedule (3). For physician integration and clinical integration, they were asked whether the item/activity was just getting started (1) to fully in place (3).

Telephone interviews were conducted with the system leaders. The same set of individuals listed for the surveys were targeted for telephone interviews that were approximately one and one-half hours long. The leaders were asked about the barriers and challenges, facilitators, better practices, and lessons learned for functional integration, physician integration, and clinical integration. These questions were also asked regarding the system's governance and management structures plus how the various system components related to one another in these areas. Representatives from all nine systems were interviewed; the actual average number of interviews per system was 4.0.

Finally, these materials were supplemented with information gathered from a related physician-system alignment study in which many of the featured systems participated. This study involved data collection using physician-level and group-level surveys as well as extensive site visits. Some of this information was drawn on in the discussion of physician-system integration in Chapter Four.

. . . . . . . . . . . . . . . . . . . . . . . . . . . . . . . . .

## Advocate Health Care

| | |
|---|---|
| Headquarters | Oak Brook, Illinois |
| Area(s) served | Greater Chicago metropolitan area |
| Total revenues | $1.6 billion combined (1997) |
| Total assets | $1.9 billion combined (1997) |
| Operating units | Has 8 owned with a total of 3,376 beds; 200 sites of care facilities including 35 Advocate Health Centers; and numerous outpatient diagnostic centers and physician office buildings throughout the Chicago area. |
| Managed care | Owns Health Direct, Inc., a managed care organization that includes an HMO and a PPO covering a combined total of 336,000 people. |

## Baylor Health Care System

| | |
|---|---|
| Headquarters | Dallas, Texas |
| Area(s) served | Dallas metropolitan area |
| Total revenues | $993.2 million (June 1998) |
| Total assets | $772.4 million (June 1998) |

| | |
|---|---|
| Operating units | Full ownership of 5 acute care hospitals (total of 1,862 licensed acute care beds), 6 senior health centers, 2 specialty hospitals, and 1 of each of the following: PPO, PHO, home health care agency, 2 ambulatory surgery center, sports medicine and research center, and durable medical equipment company; manages 4 single specialty physician group practices. |
| Managed care | Full ownership in Southwest Preferred Health Network (PPO); minority ownership in Aetna-SWHP (HMO) and North Texas Health Network. |

## Fairview Health Services

| | |
|---|---|
| Headquarters | Minneapolis, Minnesota |
| Area(s) served | Twin Cities metropolitan area and areas northeast of the Twin Cities metropolitan area |
| Total revenues | $1.0 billion (December 1997) |
| Total assets | $429.1 million (December 1997) |
| Operating units | Owned: 6 general acute care hospitals (with 1,836 total licensed beds), 20 primary care clinics, 1 skilled nursing facility, 1 home health agency, 1 ambulatory surgery center, 4 retail pharmacies, and Offshore Insurance Captive (1 unit), Healthworks (2 units), and the Institute for Athletic Medicine (21 units), 1 PHO, and 1 philanthropic foundation. |
| Managed care: | 60 percent ownership in a managed care company that manages a PPO and a long-term contracting relationship with a staff-model HMO (Health Partners) |

# Franciscan Health System

| | |
|---|---|
| Headquarters | Tacoma, Washington |
| Area(s) serve: | Pacific Northwest (Oregon and Washington State). |
| Total revenues | $21 million (1998) |
| Total assets | $262.7 million (1998) |
| Operating units: | 5 acute care hospitals, 10 nursing homes, 1 extended care facility, 8 home health care agencies, 6 durable medical equipment companies (some through joint ventures), 3 diagnostic imaging centers, 4 ambulatory surgery centers, 300 employed physicians in 3 primary care group practices, 10 PHOs, 10 philanthropic foundations, and a mobile magnetic resonance imaging multisite unit |
| Managed care | FHS does not have a system-level managed care division; managed care contracting is handled at the regional level; FHS is evaluating joint-venture opportunities and risk contracts with various HMOs in FHS—East and West markets |

# Henry Ford Health System

| | |
|---|---|
| Headquarters | Detroit, Michigan |
| Area(s) served | Detroit metropolitan area |
| Total revenues | $2.0 billion (1999) |
| Total assets | $1.8 billion (1996) |
| Operating units | Full ownership of 1 tertiary hospital (903 beds), 2 acute care community hospitals (534 total beds), 2 specialty hospitals (165 beds), 2 nursing homes, 2 skilled nursing |

facilities, 13 independent pharmacies, 27 independent laboratories, 27 diagnostic imaging centers, 4 ambulatory surgery centers, 8 IPAs, 3 PHOs, 36 ambulatory care centers offering primary and specialty care, and 1 of each of the following: home health care agency, durable medical equipment company, PPO, and dialysis company; also owns institutes or centers that conduct research on improving the process of health care delivery, including the Center for Health System Studies, Biostatistics, Research Epidemiology, and Medical Informatics), the Center for Clinical Effectiveness, and the new Center for Health Promotion and Disease Prevention

Managed care     Owns Health Alliance Plan (HAP), the largest HMO in Michigan, covering approximately 450,000 of the 950,000 HMO managed care enrollees in the Detroit metropolitan area; in addition, HAP owns Medical Value Plan), a nonprofit HMO in Toledo, Ohio, which has 35,000 members

## Mercy Health Services

Headquarters     Farmington Hills, Michigan

Area(s) served   Michigan, Iowa, Indiana, New York, Illinois and Nebraska

Total revenues   $2.5 billion (1998)

Total assets     $1.3 billion (1998)

Operating units  Majority/full ownership of 23 acute care hospitals and 1 specialty hospital, and manages an additional 12 acute care hospitals and 1 specialty hospital (total of 5,152 licensed acute care beds in the acute care hospitals owned and operated by MHS). Other units owned and operated by MHS include 17 nursing homes, 15 skilled nursing facilities, 1 home health care agency (Amicare Home Healthcare Company—with several operating units providing home health services; AHHC also provides durable medical equipment services), 11 independent pharmacies, 1 independent laboratory, 22 diagnostic imaging centers, 1 ambulatory surgery center, 12 physician/ hospital organizations, and 1 philanthropic foundation.

Managed care:    MHS subsidiary Mercy Health Plans has a total of 265,800 covered lives in Care Choices HMO, Care Choices Senior (a Medicare HMO), and Preferred Choices PPO.

## Sentara Healthcare

Headquarters     Norfolk, Virginia

Area(s) served   Southern and Eastern Shore of Virginia, northeastern North Carolina

Total revenues   $1.1 billion (December 1998)

Total assets     $1.2 billion (December 1994)

Operating units  Full or majority ownership in 4 acute care hospitals (with a total of 1,823 licensed acute care beds), 7 nursing homes, 5 ambulatory surgery centers, 4 retirement centers, 2 single specialty group practices, 2 HMOs, and 1 of each of the following: home health care agency, durable medical equipment company, independent pharmacy, and independent laboratory. Also manages 2 other single specialty group practices.

Managed care          Sentara Health Plan, a 10-site primary care
                      staff model HMO that benefits 3,000 state em-
                      ployees; Sentara Mental Health Management,
                      with over 740,000 subscribers; Sentara Direct
                      Contracting, which manages and negotiates
                      managed care contracts for Sentara Hospitals,
                      covering over 20,000 lives; also 80 percent
                      ownership in OPTIMA Health Plan, an IPA
                      model HMO covering over 245,000 members.

## Sisters of Providence

Headquarters          Seattle, Washington

Areas served          Alaska, California, Oregon, and Washington,
                      with the majority of its operating units con-
                      centrated in the latter two states.

Total revenues        $2.3 billion (December 1997)

Total assets          $2.4 billion (December 1997)

Operating units       19 acute care hospitals (3,748 licensed beds),
                      11 skilled nursing facilities (1,361 long-term
                      beds), 9 home health care agencies, 2 HMOs,
                      2 PPOs, 2 multisite primary care group
                      practices (1 in Oregon, 1 in Washington),
                      2 durable medical equipment companies,
                      1 retirement center, and 1 independent labora-
                      tory. Manages 1 skilled nursing facility, 1 home
                      care agency, and two acute care hospitals.

Managed care          100 percent ownership of the Good Health
                      Plan of Washington (an HMO with 69,290
                      members); Providence Health Care (a health
                      plan for Medicaid enrollees with 56,082 en-
                      rollees); Sound Health (a PPO with 127,432
                      covered lives); the Good Health Plan in Ore-
                      gon (an HMO with approximately 191,805

members); and Vantage (Providence Health System's Oregon PPO, with 142,822 members)

## Sutter Health

| | |
|---|---|
| Headquarters | Sacramento, California |
| Area(s) served | Sacramento, Central Valley, Bay Area, and northern California region |
| Total revenues | $2.9 billion (December 1998) |
| Total assets | $1.3 billion (December 1998) |
| Operating units | Majority or full ownership in 12 acute care hospitals (total of 5,537 licensed beds), 2 psychiatric hospitals (total of 226 beds), 4 skilled nursing facilities, 1 adult day care center, 1 home health care agency, 1 retirement center, 5 philanthropic foundations, 3 biomedical engineering centers, 2 community clinics, 1 durable medical equipment company, 5 medical foundations (which include 8 multispecialty medical groups), and 3 diagnostic imaging centers. Joint-venture interest in an outpatient surgery center with locations in four states. Partial ownership of a clinical laboratory company. |
| Managed care | Owns 100 percent of Sutter Preferred Insurance Administrators (third-party administrators with 23,726 covered lives), 100 percent of Sutter Preferred Health and Life (insurance company with 30,389 covered lives), and 75 percent of Sutter Preferred/OMNI (HMO with a total of 106,362 covered lives). Sutter Health has 252,000 covered lives under capitation contracts through partially owned and nonowned products. |

# References

Abbott, A. *The System of Professions: An Essay on the Division of Expert Labor.* Chicago: University of Chicago Press, 1988.

Ackoff, R. *The Systems Approach.* New York: Dell, 1979.

Advocate Health Care. "Strategic Priorities and Key Tactics." Internal document, Advocate Health Care, 1999.

Advisory Board. *Future Revenues: Sustainable Growth Strategies for America's Health System.* Washington, D.C.: Advisory Board, 1997.

Alexander, J. A., and Morrisey, M. A. "Hospital-Physician Integration and Hospital Costs." *Inquiry,* 1988, *25*(3), 388–402.

Alexander, J. A., and others. "An Exploratory Analysis of Market-Based Physician-Organization Arrangements." *Hospital and Health Services Administration,* 1996a, *41*(3), 311–329.

Alexander, J., and others. "Organizational Approaches to Integrated Healthcare Delivery: A Taxonomic Analysis of Physician-Organization Arrangements." *Medical Care Research and Review,* 1996b, *53*(1), 71–93.

Alexander, J. A., Zuckerman, H. S. and Pointer, D. D. "The Challenges of Governing Integrated Health Care Systems." *Health Care Management Review,* 1995, *20*(4), 69–81.

Anders, G. *Health Against Wealth.* Boston: Houghton Mifflin, 1996.

Annison, M., and Wilford, D. *Trust Matters: New Directions in Health Care Leadership.* San Francisco: Jossey-Bass, 1998.

Appleby, C. "Organized Chaos." *Hospital and Health Networks,* Jul. 20, 1997, pp. 51–52.

Argote, L. "Group and Organizational Learning Curves: Individual, System and Environmental Components." *British Journal of Social Psychology,* 1993, *32*, pp. 31–51.

Arthur Andersen and the American Hospital Association. "National Hospital Quality Improvement Survey." Knowledge Leadership Series. Issue No. 3. Chicago, 1999a.

Arthur Andersen and the American Hospital Association. *Progressive Practices in System Integration and Chronic Care Management/NCCC*. Knowledge Leadership Series, Issue No. 2. Chicago, 1999b.

Barnsley, J., Lemieux-Charles, L., and McKinney, M. M. "Integrating Learning into Integrated Delivery Systems." *Health Care Management Review*, 1998, *23*(1), 18–28.

Barr, J. L., Laufenberg, S., and Sieckman, B. L. "Creating a Vision for Your Call Center." *Health Care Information Management*, 1998, *12*(2), 71–85.

Bartling, A. C. "Integrated Delivery Systems: Fact or Fiction." *Healthcare Executive*, May–June 1995, pp. 6–11.

Bazzoli, G. J., Chan, C., and Shortell, S. "Interorganizational Strategies in the Health Industry: Effects on Hospital Financial Performance." *Best Papers, Proceedings of the Academy of Management Meetings*, Aug. 1999, B1–B6.

Bazzoli, G. J., Dynan, L., Burns, L. R., and Lindrooth, R. C. "Is Provider Capitation Working? Effects of Capitation on Integration and Hospital Cost of Care." *Medical Care*, 2000, *38*(3), 311–324.

Bazzoli, G. J., and others. "Public-Private Collaboration in Health and Human Service Delivery: Evidence from Community Partnerships." *Milbank Quarterly*, 1997, *75*(4), 533–561.

Bazzoli, G. J., and others. "A Taxonomy of Health Care Networks and Systems: Bringing Order Out of Chaos." *Health Services Research*, 1999, *33*(6), 1683–1717.

Begun, J. W., and Lippincott, R. C. *Strategic Adaptation in the Health Professions: Meeting the Challenges of Change*. San Francisco: Jossey-Bass, 1993.

Begun, J. W., and Luke, R. "Health Care Organizations and the Development of the Strategic Management Perspective." In S. Mick and others (eds.), *Innovations in Health Care Delivery: Insights for Organization Theory*. San Francisco: Jossey-Bass, 1990.

Begun, J. W., Luke, R. D., and Pointer, D. D. "Structure and Strategy in Hospital-Physician Relationships." In S. Mick and others (eds.), *Innovations in Health Care Delivery*. San Francisco: Jossey-Bass, 1990.

Beiser, M., Shore, J. H., Peters, R., and Tatum, E. "Does Community Care for the Mentally Ill Make a Difference? A Tale of Two Cities." *American Journal of Psychiatry*, 1985, *142*, 1047–1052.

Bellah, R. N., and others. *Habits of the Heart*. Berkeley: University of California Press, 1998.

Berg, K. "Specialist Ventures: New Business Partnerships with Hospitals." *Medical Network Strategy Report*, 1999, *1*, 7–11.

Berwick, D. "The Total Customer Relationship in Health Care: Broadening the Band-width." *Journal of Quality Improvement*, 1998, *23*(5), 245–250.

Berwick, D., Godfrey, A. B., and Roessner, J. *Curing Health Care*. San Francisco: Jossey-Bass, 1990.

Berwick, D., and Kilo, C. M. "Idealized Design of Clinical Office Practice: An Interview with Donald Berwick and Charles Kilo of the Institute for Healthcare Improvement." *Managed Care Quarterly*, 1999, *7*(4), 62–69.

Blumenthal, D., and Kilo, C. M. "A Report Card on Continuous Quality Improvement." *Milbank Quarterly*, 1998, *76*(4), 625–648.

Blumenthal, D., and Laffel, G. "The Case for Using Industrial Quality Management Science in Health Care Organizations." *Journal of the American Medical Association*, 1989, *262*, 2669–2873.

Bodenheimer, T. "The American Health Care System—Physicians and the Changing Medical Marketplace." *New England Journal of Medicine*, 1999, *340*(7), 584–588.

Bogue, R. J., Antia, M., Harmata, R., and Hall, C. H. "Community Experiments in Action: Developing Community-defined Models for Reconfiguring Health Care Delivery." *Journal of Health Politics, Policy and Law*, 1997, *22*, 1051–1076.

Bogue, R. J., and Hall, C. H., Jr. (eds.). *Health Network Innovations: How 20 Communities Are Improving Their Systems Through Collaboration*. Chicago: American Hospital Publisher, 1997.

Bollinger, J. "Effective Physician Integration Strategy." *Healthcare Strategic Management*, Jul. 1999, pp. 18–20.

Boult, C., and Pacala, J. T. "Integrating Health Care for Older Populations." *American Journal of Managed Care*, 1999, *5*(1), 45–52.

Bower, K. A. "Clinically Integrated Delivery Systems and Case Management." In M. Tonges (ed.), *Clinical Integration: Strategies and Practices for Organized Delivery Systems*. San Francisco: Jossey-Bass, 1998.

Bradford, D., and Cohen, A. R. *Managing for Excellence*. New York: Wiley, 1984.

Bringewatt, R. J. "The Future Role of Integrated Delivery System in Serving Older Adults." Minnesota Senior Health Options, 1998 Annual Educational Forum, Jan. 22, 1999, p. 20.

Burns, L. R., Cacciamani, J., Clement, J., and Aquino, W. "The Fall of the House of AHERF: The Allegheny Bankruptcy." *Health Affairs*, 2000, *19*(1), 7–41.

Burns, L. R., and Robinson, J. C. "Physician Practice Management Companies: Implications for Hospital-based Integrated Delivery Systems." *Frontiers of Health Services Management*, 1997, *14*(2), 3–35.

Burns, L. R., and Thorpe, D. P. "Trends and Models in Physician-Hospital Organization." *Health Care Management Review*, 1993, *18*(4), 7–20.

Burns, L. R., and others. "Physician Alignment with Organized Delivery Systems," working paper, University of Pennsylvania, 2000.

Burns, L. R., and Thorpe, D. P. "Why Provider-Sponsored Health Plans Don't Work." Healthcare Financial Management, forthcoming.

Burton, T. M. "An HMO Checks up on Its Doctors' Care and Is Disturbed Itself." *Wall Street Journal*, Aug. 23, 1999, p. 1.

Carey, R. G., and Teeters, J .L. "CQI Case Study: Reducing Medication Errors." *Joint Commission Journal on Quality Improvement*, 1995, *21*(5), 232–237.

"Case Study: Using the National Chronic Care Consortium's (NCCC's) Self-assessment for Systems Integration (SASI) Tool—The Fairview Experience." *Integrated Patient Care*, 1997, *1*(2), pp. 1, 10–12.

Center for the Advancement of Health. *Patients as Effective Collaborators in Managing Chronic Conditions*. New York: Milbank Memorial Fund, 1999.

Champy, J., and Hammer, M. *Reengineering the Corporation: A Manifesto for Business Revolution*. New York: Harper, 1993.

Chandler, A. D. *Strategy and Structure: Chapters in the History of the Industrial Enterprise*. Cambridge, Mass.: MIT Press, 1962.

Charns, M. P. and Tewksbury, L .J. *Collaborative Management in Health Care: Implementing the Integrated Organization*. San Francisco: Jossey-Bass, 1993.

Chassin, M. R. "Is Health Care Ready for Six Sigma Quality?" *Milbank Quarterly*, 1998, *76*(4), 565–591.

Chassin, M. R., Galvin, R. W., and the National Roundtable on Health Care Quality. "The Urgent Need to Improve Health Care Quality." *Journal of the American Medical Association*, 1998, *280*, 1000–1005.

Churchman, C. W. *Redesigning the Future: A Systems Approach to Societal Problems*. New York: Wiley, 1974.

Cleary, P. D., and Edgman, S. "Health Care Quality: Incorporating Consumer Perspectives." *Journal of the American Medical Association*, 1998, *278*, 1608–1612.

Cleary, P. D., and McNeil, B. J. "Patient Satisfaction as an Indicator of Quality Care." *Inquiry*, 1988, *25*, 25–36.

Coberly, S. "Chronic Care Clinics: Group Health Cooperative of Puget Sound." In S. Coberly (ed.), *Managing Care, Operations and Performance: Innovations in Organized Systems of Care*. Washington, D.C.: Washington Business Group on Health, 1998.

Coddington, D. C., Moore, K. D., and Fischer, E. A. *Integrated Health Care: Reorganizing the Physician, Hospital, Health Plan Relationship*. Englewood, Colo.: Center for Research in Ambulatory Health Care Administration, MGMA, 1994.

Coile, R. C. *Millennium Management: Better, Faster, Cheaper Strategies for Managing 21st Century Health Care Organizations*. Chicago: Health Administration Press, 1999.

Conrad, D. "Coordinating Patient Care Services in Regional Health Systems: The Challenge of Clinical Integration." *Hospital and Health Services Administration*, 1993, *38*(4), 491–508.

Conrad, D. A., and Shortell, S. M. "Integrated Health Systems: Promise and Performance." *Frontiers of Health Services Management*, 1996, *13*, 345–354.

Conrad, D. T., and others. "Managing Care, Incentives, and Information: An Exploratory Look Inside the Black Box of Hospital Efficiency." *Health Services Research*, 1996, *31*(3), 235–259.

D'Aunno, T. A., and Zuckerman, H. S. "The Life Cycle of Organization Federations." *Academy of Management Review*, 1987, *12*(3), 534–545.

Darby, M. "Coordinating Care in an Integrated Delivery System." *Quality Letter*, 1999, *11*(7), 2–11.

Deming, W. E. *Out of the Crisis*. Cambridge, Mass.: Center for Advanced Engineering Study, Massachusetts Institute of Technology, 1986.

Devers, K. J., and others. "Implementing Organized Delivery Systems: An Integration Scorecard." *Health Care Management Review*, 1994, *19*(3), 7–20.

Dorenfest, S. I. and Sheldon, I. *H.C.I.S. Market Review*. Chicago: Dorenfest and Associates, Ltd., 1995.

Drucker, P. "The Theory of the Business." *Harvard Business Review*, Sept.–Oct. 1994, pp. 95–104.

Drucker, P. "Why Management Matters." *Harvard Business Review*, Oct. 5, 1998.

Dunham, N. C., Kindig, D. A., and Schulz, R. "The Value of the Physician Executive Role to Organizational Effectiveness and Performance." *Health Care Management Review*, 1994, *19*(4), 54–63.

Dynan, L., Bazzoli, G. and Burns, L. "Assessing the Extent to Integration Achieved Through Physician-Hospital Arrangements." *Journal of Healthcare Management*, 1998, *43*, 242–262.

Eddy, C. "A Time for Reflection: Providers Rethink Plan Ownership." *Medical Network Strategy Report*, 1999, B(2), 6.

Eichhorn, J. H. "Prevention of Intraoperative Anesthesia Accidents and Related Severe Injury Through Safety Monitoring." *Anesthesiology*, 1989, *70*(4), 572–577.

Eisenberg, D., and others. "Trends in Alternative Medicine Use in the United States, 1990–1997." *Journal of the American Medical Association*, 1998, *280*(11), 1569–1575.

Eisenhardt, K. M., and Brown, S. "Patching: Restitching Business Portfolios in Dynamic Markets." *Harvard Business Review*, May-June 1999, 75–85.

Emanuel, E. J., and Emanuel, L. L. "What Is Accountability in Health Care?" *Annals of Internal Medicine*, 1996, *124*, 229–239.

Etzioni, A. "Communitarian Elements in Select Works of Martin Buber." *Journal of Value Inquiry*, 1999, *33*(2), 151–169.

Evans, R., Barer, M., and Marmor, T. *Why Are Some People Healthy and Others Not? The Determinants of Health of Populations*. New York: Aldine de Gruyter, 1994.

Farrell, J. P. "Reshaping Governance: The Hay Group's Study." *Trustee*, 1995, *48*(6), 22–24.

Flexner, A. *Medical Education in the United States and Canada*. Bulletin No. 4. New York: Carnegie Foundation for the Advancement of Teaching, 1910.

Fowler, F., and Stokes, J. "Case Management from Multi-Provider Systems." *Case Manager*, 1996, *7*(5), 63–69.

Freidson, E. *Professional Dominance: The Social Structure of Medical Care*. New York: Atherton Press, 1970a.

Freidson, E. *Profession of Medicine*. New York: HarperCollins, 1970b.

Galvin, R. "What Do Employers Mean by Value?" *Integrated Healthcare Report*, Oct. 1998, pp. 1–10.

Gillies, R. R., and others. "Conceptualizing and Measuring Integration: Findings from the Health Systems Integration Study." *Hospital and Health Services Administration*, 1993, *38*(4), 467–489.

Goes, J. B., and Zhan, L. L. "The Effects of Hospital-Physician Integration Strategies on Hospital Financial Performance." *Health Services Research*, 1995, *30*(4), 507–530.

Gold, M. R., Franks, P., McCoy, K. I., and Fryback, D. G. "Toward Consistency in Cost-Utility Analyses: Using National Measures to Creation-Specific Values." *Medical Care*, 1998, *36*(6), 778–792.

Goldsmith, J. C. "Driving the Nitroglycerin Truck." *Healthcare Forum Journal*, Mar.–Apr. 1993, pp. 36–44.

Goldsmith, J. C. "The Elusive Logic of Integration." *Health Forum Journal*, 1994, *37*(5), 26–31.

Goldsmith, J. C. "Risk and Responsibility: The Evolution of Health Care Payment." In Institute of Medicine, *2020 Vision Health in the 21st Century*. Washington, D.C.: National Academy Press, 1996.

Goldsmith, J. C. "Integration Reconsidered: Five Strategies for Improved Performance." *Healthcare Strategist*, 1998a, *2*, 1–8.

Goldsmith, J. C. "Operation Restore Human Values." *Hospitals and Health Networks*, Jul. 5, 1998b, pp. 74–76.

Gosfield, A. G. *Quality and Clinical Culture: The Critical Role of Physicians in Accountable Healthcare Organizations*. Chicago: Department of Organized Medical Staff Services, American Medical Association, 1998.

Grant, L. "Your Customers Are Telling the Truth." *Fortune*, Feb. 1, 1998, pp. 164–165.

Greenhouse, S. "Angered by HMO's Treatment, More Doctors Are Joining Unions." *New York Times*, Feb. 4, 1999, pp. A1, A25.

Griffith, J. R. "The Infrastructure of Integrated Delivery Systems." *Healthcare Executive*, May–June 1995, pp. 12–17.

Griffith, J. R., Sahney, V. K., and Mohr, R. A. *Reengineering Health Care: Building on CQI*. Ann Arbor, Mich.: Health Administration Press, 1995.

Grumbach, K., and others. "Resolving the Gatekeeper Conundrum: What Patients Value in Primary Care and Referrals to Specialists." *Journal of the American Medical Association*, Jul. 21, 1999, pp. 261–266.

Haas-Wilson, D., and Gaynor, M. "Increasing Consolidation in Healthcare Markets: What Are the Anti-Trust Policy Implications?" *Health Services Research*, 1998, *33*(5), 1477–1494.

Hafferty, F. W., and Light, D. W. "Professional Dynamics and the Changing Nature of Medical Work." *Journal of Health and Social Behavior*, 1995, *36*, 132–153.

Hall, G., Rosenthal, J., and Wade, J. "How to Make Reengineering Really Work." *Harvard Business Review*, Nov.–Dec. 1993, pp. 119–131.

Handy, C. *The Age of Paradox*. Boston: Harvard Business School Press, 1994.

Harrigan, K. R. *Strategies for Declining Businesses*. Lexington, Mass.: Lexington Books, 1980.

Harrington, C., Lynch, M., and Newcomer, R. J. "Medical Services in Social Health Maintenance Organizations." *Gerontologist*, 1993, *33*, 790–800.

Harrington, C., and Newcomer, R. J. "Social Health Maintenance Organization's Service Use and Cost, 1985-1989." *Health Care Financing Review*, 1991, *12*, 37–52.

Havighurst, L. A. "A Union Answer, the growing dominance of managed care—with reduced pay and job measures—has led some physicians to search for strength in numbers." *American Medical News*, Jan. 11, 1999.

Havlicek, P. *Medical Group Practices in the U.S.: A Survey of Practice Characteristics*. Chicago: American Medical Association, 1999.

Health Care Advisory Board. *TQM: Directory of Hospital Projects*. Washington, D.C.: Advisory Board Company, 1992.

Health Care Advisory Board. *Twin Cities Report*. Washington, D.C.: Health Care Advisory Board, 1998.

Hellinger, F. J. "Anti-trust Enforcement in the Health Care Industry: The Expanding Scope of State Activity." *Health Services Research*, 1998, *33*(5), 1537–1562.

Henry Ford Health System. *Cost-Effectiveness of Integrated Group Practice: A Case Study*. Detroit, Mich.: Henry Ford Medical Group, 1993.

Herzlinger, R. *Market Driven Health Care*. Reading, Mass.: Addison-Wesley, 1996.

Hill, J., and Wild, J. "Survey Provides Data on Practice Acquisition Activity." *Healthcare Financial Management*, Sept. 1995, 54–71.

Huber, G. P., and Glick, W. H. *Organizational Change and Redesign: Ideas and Insights for Improving Performance*. New York: Oxford University Press, 1993.

Hughes, E. "The Ascendancy of Management: National Health Care Reform, Managed Competition and Its Implications for Physician Executives." In W. Curry (ed.), *New Leadership in Health Care Management: The Physician Executive II*. Tampa, Fla.: American College of Physician Executives, 1994.

Hunt, R. S. "Overcoming Barriers to Integrated Health Delivery." *Frontiers of Health Services Management*, 1996, *13*(1), 50–52.

Iezzoni, L. Risk *Adjustment for Measuring Health Care Outcomes*. Ann Arbor, Mich.: Health Administration Press, 1994.

"Innovations and Issues in Clinical Integration: Improving Systems for MSHO Clients." Minnesota Senior Health Options, Annual Educational Forum, Minneapolis, 1997.

Institute for Health and Aging. *Chronic Care in America: A 21st Century Challenge*. San Francisco: Institute for University of California, 1996.

Institute of Medicine. *Committee Designing the 21st Century Health System*. Washington, D.C.: National Academy Press, 2000a.

Institute of Medicine. *To Err Is Human: Building a Safer Health System*. Washington, D.C.: National Academy Press, 2000b.

*Internet News*, Apr. 1, 1999.

Juran, J. *Juran on Leadership for Quality: An Executive*. New York: Free Press, 1989.

Kane, R. L., and others. "S/HMO The Second Generation: Building on the Experience of the First Social Health Maintenance Organization Demonstrations." *Journal of the American Geriatric Society*, 1997, *45*, 101–107.

Kanter, R. M. "Collaborative Advantage: The Art of Alliances." *Harvard Business Review*, July-Aug. 1994, pp. 96–108.

Kaplan, R. S., and Norton, D. P. "The Balanced Scorecard: Measures that Drive Performance." *Harvard Business Review*, Jan.–Feb. 1992, pp. 71–79.

Kaplan, R. S., and Norton, D. P. "Putting the Balanced Scorecard to Work." *Harvard Business Review*, Sept.–Oct. 1993, pp. 134–137.

Kassirer, J. P. "Managing Care—Should We Adopt a New Ethic?" *New England Journal of Medicine*, 1998, 339(6), 397–398.

Kimberly, J. *The Organizational Life Cycle*. San Francisco: Jossey-Bass, 1980.

Kind, P. C., Gudex, C., and Dolan, P. "Practical and Methodological Experience with the Development of the EuroQuol." In G. L. Albrecht (ed.), *Quality of Life in Health Care: Advances in Medical Sociology*. Greenwich, Conn.: JAI Press, 1994.

Kindig, D. A. *Purchasing Population Health: Paying for Results*. Ann Arbor: University of Michigan Press, 1997.

Kindig, D. A. "Purchasing Population Health: Aligning Financial Incentives to Improve Health Outcomes." *Health Services Research*, 1998, 33(2), 223–242.

Klein, S. A. "AMA to Establish National Collective Bargaining Unit." *American Medical News*, 1999, 42(5) [http://www.ama-assn.org/sci-pubs/msjama/articles/vol_281/no_27/union.htm].

Kleinke, J. D. *Bleeding Edge: The Business of Health Care in the New Century*. Gaithersburg, Md.: Aspen, 1998.

Kovner, A. R., Ritvo, R. A., and Holland, T. P. "Board Development in Two Hospitals: Lessons from a Demonstration." *Hospital and Health Services Administration*, 1997, 42(1), 87–99.

Kralovec, J. "The Critical Role Information Systems Play in Reengineering Efforts." *Quality Letter*, 1994, 6(7), 11–13.

Kreuter, M., and Lezin, N. *Are Consortia/Collaboratives Effective in Changing Health Status and Health Systems? A Critical Review of the Literature*. (Prepared for the Health Resources and Service Administration Office of Planning, Evaluation, and Legislation [OPEL]. Atlanta: Health 2000, 1998.

Kuttner, R. "Physician-Operated Networks and the New Anti-Trust Guidelines." *New England Journal of Medicine*, 1997, 336, 386–391.

Langley, K., and others. *The Improvement Guide*. San Francisco: Jossey-Bass, 1996.

Leatt, P., and Leggatt, S. G. "Governing Integrated Health Delivery Systems: Meeting Accountability Requirements." *Healthcare Management Forum*, Winter 1997, pp. 12–25.

Lehman, A. F., and others. "Continuity of Care in Client Outcomes." *Milbank Quarterly*, 1994, 72, 105–122.

Libby, D. L., and others. *Wisconsin Population Health Check-up*. Madison: Wisconsin Network for Health Policy Research, University of Wisconsin School of Medicine, 1997.

Liebenluft, R. F. "Attempts to Level the Playing Field-Developments in HMO Merger Enforcements, Anti-Trust Exemptions, and Physician Unions." *Health Law Digest*, 1999, 23, 3–11.

Light, D. "Countervailing Power; The Changing Character of the Medical Profession in the United States." In F. Hafferty and J. McKinley (eds.), *The Changing Character of the Medical Profession: An International Perspective*, New York: Oxford University Press, 1993.

Lind, E. A., and Tyler, T. R. *Social Psychology of Procedural Justice*. New York: Plenum, 1988.

Lunn, J. N., and Devlin, H. B. "Lessons From the Confidential Enquiry into Perioperative Deaths in Three NHS Regions." *Lancet*, Dec. 12, 1987, pp. 1384–1387.

Manton, K. G., and others. "Social-Health Maintenance Organizations and Fee-for-Service Outcomes over Time." *Health Care Financing Review*, 1993, *15*, 173–202.

McKnight, J. *The Careless Society: Community and Its Counterfeits*. New York: Basic Books, 1995.

Menke, T. J. "The Effects of Chain Membership on Hospital Costs." *Health Services Research*, 1997, *32*(2), 177–196.

Millenson, M. *Demanding Medical Excellence*. Chicago: University of Chicago Press, 1997.

Miller, R., Lipton, H., and Duke, K. S. *Health System Change in the Greater Sacramento Area*. Sacramento, Calif.: Sierra Health Foundation, 1997.

Mintzberg, H., and Glouberman, S. "Managing the Care of Health and the Care of Disease Part 2: Integration." Working Paper, McGill University, Feb. 1997.

Missouri Department of Health. *"Show Me. . ."*: *Buyer's Guide: Managed Care Plans*. Jefferson City, Mo.: Missouri Department of Health, 1998.

Mittman, R., and Cain, M. *The Future of the Internet in Health Care: A Five-Year Forecast*. Menlo Park, Calif.: Institute for the Future, and Oakland, Calif.: California Health Foundation, 1999.

Molinari, C., Alexander, J., Morlock, L., and Lyles, C. A. "Does the Hospital Board Need a Doctor? The Influence of Physician Board Participation on Hospital Financial Performance." *Medical Care*, 1995, *33*(2), 170–185.

Morlock, L., and Alexander, J. "Models of Governance in Multihospital Systems: Implications for Hospital and System-Level Decision-Making." *Medical Care*, 1986, *24*(12), 1118–1135.

Morrisey, M., Alexander, J. A., Burns, L., and Johnson, V. "Managed Care and Physician-Hospital Integration." *Health Affairs*, 1996, *15*(4), 62–73.

Morrisey, M. A., Alexander, J. A., Burns, L. R., and Johnson, V. "The Effects of Managed Care on Physicians and Clinical Integration in Hospitals." *Medical Care*, 1999, *37*(4), 350–361.

Mycek, S. "Leadership for a Healthy 21st Century." *Health Care Forum Journal*, 1998, *41*(4), 26–30.

Nelson, E. C., and others. "Report Cards or Instrument Panels: Who Needs What?" *Joint Commission Journal of Quality Improvement*, 1995, *21*(4), 155–166.

Newcomer R., Harrington C., and Friedlob, A. "Social Health Maintenance Organizations: Assessing Their Initial Experience." *Health Services Research*, 1990, *25*(3), 425–454.

O'Brien, J. L., and others. "An Integrative Model for Organization-wide Quality Improvement: Lessons from the Field." *Quality Management in Health Care*, 1995, *3*(4), 19–30.

Ohsfeldt, R. L., Morrisey, M. A., Nelson, L. J., and Johnson, V. "The Spread of State Any Willing Provider Laws." *Health Services Research*, 1998, *33*(5), 1537–1562.

Orkin, F. W. "Patient Monitoring During Anesthesia as an Exercise in Technology Assessment." In L. J. Saidman and N. T. Smith (eds.), *Monitoring in Anesthesia* (3rd ed.). London: Butterworth-Heineman, 1993.

Orlikoff, J. E. "From Hospital to Health System Governance: The Changing Characteristics of Boards." *Healthcare Executive*, Sept-Oct. 1997, *12*(5), 14–18.

Orlikoff, J. E. "Ensuring Board Effectiveness: It Could Be As Simple As Changing Your Board Structure." *Healthcare Executive*, 1998, *13*(5), 12–16.

Orlikoff, J. E., and Totten, M. K. "Getting from Here to There." *Trustee*, 1996, *49*(6), 16–20.

Patton, M. Q. "The Program's Theory of Action: Evaluating Causal Linkages." In *Utilization-Focused Evaluation*. Thousand Oaks, Calif.: Sage, 1978.

Pauly, M. V. *Doctors and Their Workshops: Economic Models of Physician Behavior.* Chicago: University of Chicago Press, 1980.

Perkins, K. D. "Berkeley Health Center Gives Peek at the Future." *San Francisco Examiner*, July 11, 1999, p. D-2.

Planck, M. Wissenschaftliche Selbstbiographie. Leipzig: Johann Ambrosius Barth Verlag, 1948.

Pointer, D. D., Alexander, J. A., and Zuckerman, H. S. "Loosening the Gordian Knot of Governance in Integrated Health Care Delivery Systems." *Frontiers of Health Services Management*, 1995, *11*(3), 3–37.

Porter, A., Van Cleave, B., and Milobowski, L. "Clinical Integration: An Interdisciplinary Approach to a System Priority." *Nursing Administration Quarterly*, 1996, *20*(2), 65–73.

Povar, G., and Shortell, S. M. "The Function of an Umbrella Organization for Effectively Functioning Micro Systems." Draft Report for the Institute of Medicine Sub-Committee on the Quality of Health Care in America, Washington, D.C., Apr. 1999.

Prahalad, C. K., and Hamel, G. "The Core Competence of the Corporation." *Harvard Business Review*, May-June 1990, pp. 79–91.

President's Advisory Commission on Consumer Protection and Quality in the Health Care Industry. *Quality First: Better Health Care for All Americans*. Washington, D.C.: U.S. Government Printing Office, 1998.

Putnam, R. D. *Making Democracy Work*. Princeton, N.J.: Princeton University Press, 1993.

Quinn, J. B. *Intelligent Enterprise*. New York: Free Press, 1992.

Reinertsen, J. "Living Guidelines." *Healthcare Forum Journal*, Nov.–Dec. 1994, pp. 58–59.

Relman, A. S. "Assessment and Accountability: The Third Revolution in Medical Care." *New England Journal of Medicine*, Nov. 3, 1988, pp. 1220–1222.

Robert Wood Johnson Foundation. *Improving Quality Illness Care Evaluation*. Santa Monica, Calif.: Rand Corporation, and Berkeley: University of California, Berkeley, 2000.

Robine, J. M. "Distinguishing Health Expectancies and Health Adjusted Life Expectancies from Quality Adjusted Life Years," *American Journal of Public Health*, 1993, 83(6), 797–798.

Robine, J. M., and Ritchie, K. "Health Life Expectancy: Evaluation of Global Indicators of Change in Population Health." *British Medicine Journal*, 1991, *302*, 457–460.

Robinson, J. C. "Physician-Hospital Integration and the Economic Theory of the Firm." *Medical Care Research and Review*, 1997, 54(1), 3–24.

Robinson, J. C. "Blended Payment Methods in Physician Organizations Under Managed Care." *JAMA*, October 6, 1999a, *282*, 1258-1263.

Robinson, J. C. *The Corporate Practice of Medicine*. Berkeley: University of California Press, 1999b.

Rosenheck, R., Frisman, L., and Kasprow, W. "Improving Access to Disability Benefits Among Homeless Persons with Mental Illness: An Agency-Specific Approach to Services Integration." *American Journal of Public Health*, 1999, 89(4), 524–528.

Rosenheck, R., and others. "Service System Integration, Access to Services and Housing Outcomes in a Program for Homeless Persons with Severe Mental Illness." *American Journal of Public Health*, 1998, 88, 1610–1615.

Ross, A. F., and Tinker, J. H. "Anesthesia Risk." In R. D. Miller (ed.), *Anesthesia* (4th ed.). New York: Churchill-Livingston, 1994.

Ross, P. A., Mackey, L. G., and Herrick, R. *Creating a Longitudinal Record of Health Service Use for Coordinated Care Clients*. Victoria, Australia: Southern Health Network, 1998.

Rundall, T. G., Starkweather, D. B., and Norrish, B. R. *After Restructuring: Empowerment Strategies at Work in America's Hospitals*. San Francisco: Jossey-Bass, 1998.

Sahney, V. K., and Warden, G. L. "The Quest for Quality and Productivity in Health Services." *Frontiers of Health Services Management*, 1991, 7(4), 2–40.

Schauffler, H. H., and Brown, E. R. *The State of Health Insurance in California*. Berkeley: Center for Health and Public Policy Studies, University of California, Berkeley, 1999.

Schauffler, H. H., Brown, C., and Milstein, A. "Raising the Bar: The Use of Performance Indicators by the Pacific Group on Health." *Health Affairs*, 1999, 18(2), 134–142.

Scheffler, R. M. "Physician Collective Bargaining: A Turning Point in U.S. Medicine." *Journal of Health Policy, Politics, and Law*, 1999, 24(5), 1071–1076.

Scherger, J., and Nelson, G. *Concept Paper: Beyond Visit-Based Practice—New Models of Practice Delivery*. Interim Report, Institute of Medicine Sub-Committee on Quality of Health Care in America, May 31, 1999.

Schlesinger, M. "Paradigms Lost: The Persistent Search for Community in U.S. Health Policy." *Journal of Health Policy, Politics and Law*, August 22, 1997, pp. 37–92.

Schuster, M. A., McGlynn, E. A., and Brook, R. H. "How Good Is the Quality of Health Care in the United States?" *Milbank Quarterly*, 1998, 76(4), 517–563.

Scott, W. R. "Managing Professional Work: Three Models of Control for Health Organizations." *Health Services Research*, 1982, 17(3), 213–240.

Senge, P. *The Fifth Discipline: The Art and Practice of the Learning Organization*. New York: Doubleday, 1990.

Shalowitz, J. I. Presentations for Executive Education Program, Allen Center, Northwestern University, 1994.

Shortell, S. M. *Effective Hospital-Physician Relationships*. Ann Arbor, Mich.: Health Administration Press, 1991.

Shortell, S. M., Bennett, C. L., and Byck, G. R. "Assessing the Impact of Continuing Quality Improvement on Clinical Practice: What It Will Take to Accelerate Progress." *Milbank Quarterly*, 1998, 76(4).

Shortell, S. M., Gillies, R. R., and Anderson, D. "The New World of Managed Care: Creating Organized Delivery Systems." *Health Affairs*, Winter 1994, pp. 46–64.

Shortell, S. M., Gillies, R., and Devers, K. J. "Reinventing the American Hospital." *Milbank Quarterly*, 1995, 73(2), 131–160.

Shortell, S. M., and others. "Creating Organized Delivery Systems: The Barriers and Facilitators." *Hospital and Health Services Administration*, 1993, 38(4), 447–466.

Shortell, S. M., and others. *Remaking Health Care in America: Building Organized Delivery Systems*. San Francisco: Jossey-Bass, 1996.

Shortell, S. M., Waters, T., Clarke, K. W., and Budetti, P. P. "Physicians as Double Agents: Maintaining Trust in an Era of Multiple Accountabilities." *Journal of the American Medical Association*, Sept. 23–30, 1998, pp. 1102–1108.

Shortell, S. M., and others. "Implementing Evidence-Based Medicine: The Role of Compensation Incentives and Culture in Physician Organizations." Working Paper, Division of Health Policy and Management and Center for Health Management Studies, University of California, Berkeley, 2000.

Simons, R. *Levers of Control, How Managers Use Innovative Controls Systems to Drive Strategic Renewal*. Boston: Harvard Business School Press, 1995.

"Single Specialty Carve Outs: A Threat to Integrated Care?" *Medical Network Strategy Report*, 1999, 8(3), 1–8.

Sirio, C. A., and Harper, D. "Designing the Optimal Health Assessment System: the Cleveland Quality Choice (CHQC)." *American Journal of Medical Quality*, 1996, 11(1), S66–69.

Siu, A. L., and others. "Choosing Quality of Care Measures Based on the Expected Impact of Improved Care of Health." *Health Services Research*, 1992, 27(5), 619–650.

Snail, T. S. "The Effects of Hospital Contracting for Physician Services on Hospital Performance." Unpublished doctoral dissertation, University of California, Berkeley, 1999.

Snail, T. S., and Robinson, J. C. "Organizational Diversification in the American Hospital." *Annual Review of Public Health*, 1998, 19, 417–453.

Stalk, G., Evans, P., and Shulman, L. "Competing on Capabilities: The New Rules of Corporate Strategy." *Harvard Business Review*, March-Apr. 1992, pp. 57–69.

Starr, P. *The Social Transformation of American Medicine*. New York: Basic Books, 1983.

Stevens, R. *American Medicine and the Public Interest*. New Haven, Conn.: Yale University Press, 1971.

Taylor, F. *Scientific Management*. New York: Harper & Row, 1947.

Teece, D. J. "The Market for Know-How and the Efficient International Transfer of Technology." *Annals of the American Association of Political and Social Sciences*, Nov. 1981, pp. 81–86.

Teece, D. J. "Capturing Value from Knowledge Assets: The New Economy, Markets for Know-How, and Intangible Assets." *California Management Review*, 1998, 40(3), 55–78.

Thompson, J. D. *Organizations in Action*. New York: McGraw-Hill, 1967.

Tyson, L. D. "HMO's: A Good Idea That Could Get a Lot Better." *Business Week*, Aug. 9, 1999, p. 20.

U.S. Public Health Service. *Healthy People 2000. National Health Promotion and Disease Prevention Objectives*. Washington, D.C.: U.S. Department of Health and Human Services, 1991.

U.S. Public Health Service. *Healthy People 2010. Understanding and Improving Health*. Washington, D.C.: U.S. Department of Health and Human Services, 2000.

VanDeusen Lukas, C., and Simon, B. "Structure of Integrating Systems." *Transition Watch*, Spring 1998, pp. 1–3.

Wachter, R. M. "An Introduction to the Hospitalist Model." *Annals of Internal Medicine*, 1999, *130*(4, part 2), 338–342.

Wachter, R. M., and Goldman, L. "The Emerging Role of 'Hospitalists' in the American Health Care System." *New England Journal of Medicine*, 1996, *335*(7), 514–517.

Wagner, E., and others. "A Survey of Leading Chronic Disease Management Programs: Are They Consistent with the Literature?" *Managed Care Quarterly*, 1999, *7*(3), 56–66. Seattle, Wash.: MacColl Center for Innovation and Health Promotion.

Walston, S. L., and Bogue, R. J. "The Effects of Reengineering: Fad or Competitive Factor?" *Journal of Healthcare Management*, 1999, *44*(6), 456–474.

Walston, S. L., Kimberly, J., and Burns, L. R. "Owned Vertical Integration and Health Care: Promise and Performance." *Health Care Management Review*, 1996, *21*(1), 83–92.

Waters, T. M., and others. "Factors Associated with Physician Involvement in Care Management." Working paper, Institute for Health Services and Policy Research, Northwestern University, 2000.

Wegner, D. M. "Transactive Memory: A Contemporary Analysis of the Group Mind." In B. Mullen and G. R. Goethals (eds.), *Theories of Group Behavior*. Hillsdale, N.J.: Erlbaum, 1986.

Wells, K. B., and others. "Detection of Depressive Disorder for Patients Receiving Prepaid or Fee-for-Service Care." *Journal of the American Medical Association*, 1989, *262*, 3298–3302.

Wennberg, J. (ed.). *The Dartmouth Atlas of Health Care*. Chicago: American Hospital Publication, 1999.

Whitelaw, M. A., and Warden, G. L. "Reexamining the Delivery System as Part of Medical Reform." *Health Affairs*, 1999, *8*(1), 132–143.

Wilensky, G. R. "Integrated Patient Care and The Future of Health Care." National Chronic Care Consortium Special Address, Dec. 9, 1997.

Wilkinson, R., Kawachi, I., and Kennedy, B. "Mortality: The Social Environment, Crime and Violence." In M. Bartley, D. Blaine, and G. Davey Smith (eds.), *Sociology of Health Inequalities*. Oxford: Blackwell, 1998.

Williams, A. "Ethics and Efficiency in the Provision of Health Care." In J. M. Bell and S. Mendus (eds.), *Philosophy and Medical Welfare*. New York: Cambridge University Press, 1988.

Williams, A. "QALY's Ethics: A Health Economist's Perspective." *Social Science and Medicine*, 1996, *43*(12), 1795–1804.

Williams, E. S., and others. "Physician, Practice, and Patient Characteristics Related to Physician Physical Mental Health: Results from the Physician Work Life Survey." Paper presented at the University of California, Berkeley Organizations Conference, Berkeley, Calif., June 10, 1999.

Williams, J. B. "Guidelines for Managing Integration." *Health Care Forum Journal*, Mar.–Apr. 1992, pp. 39–47.

Williamson, O. E. *Markets and Hierarchies, Analysis and Antitrust Implications: A Study in the Economics of Internal Organization*. New York: Free Press, 1975.

Williamson, O. E. "The Economics of Organization: The Transaction Cost Approach." *American Journal of Sociology*, 1981, *87*, 547.

Williamson, O. E. *The Economic Institutions of Capitalism: Firms, Markets, Relational Contracting*. New York: Free Press, 1985.

Williamson, O. E., and Ouchi, W. G. "The Markets and Hierarchies: Program of Research, Origins, Implications, Prospects." In W. Joyce and A. Van de Ven (eds.), *Organizational Design*. New York: Wiley, 1981.

Wong, B. "Population-Based Chronic Care and Adverse Risk Selection: Resolving the Conflict." [Interview.] *Quality Letter for Healthcare Leaders*, 1998, *10*(2), 11–14.

Zajac, E. J., D'Aunno, T. A., and Burns, L. R. "Managing Strategic Alliances." In S. M. Shortell and A. D. Kaluzny (eds.), *Health Care Management: Organization Design and Behavior* (4th ed.). Albany, N.Y.: ITP-Delmar, 2000.

Zelman, W. A. *The Changing Health Care Marketplace*. San Francisco: Jossey-Bass, 1996.

Zuckerman, H. S., and others. "Physicians and Organizations: Strange Bedfellows or a Marriage Made in Heaven?" *Frontiers of Health Services Management*, 1998, *14*, 3–34.

# Name Index

# Subject Index